The Logic Engine

Rebuilding Human Thought in the Age of Artificial Intelligence

How to Think Clearly, See Opportunity, and Build Wealth as the World Rewrites Itself

First Edition: March 2026
ISBN: 978-1-966035-02-2
Published by Elite Nutrition Research
EliteNutritionResearch.com

Disclaimer: This book is for informational purposes only. The author and publisher make no representations or warranties with respect to the accuracy or completeness of the contents of this book and disclaim all warranties, including without limitation warranties of fi tness for a particular purpose. The advice and strategies contained herein may not be suitable for every individual. The author and publisher shall not be liable for any loss or damage, including but not limited to special, incidental, consequential, or other damages.

Medical Disclaimer:
This book is intended for informational purposes only and is not a substitute for professional medical advice, diagnosis, or treatment. The content provided is based on the author's research, knowledge, and personal opinions. Always seek the advice of your physician or other qualifi ed health provider with any questions you may have regarding a medical condition. Never disregard professional medical advice or delay in seeking it because of something you have read in this book.

The author and publisher are not responsible for any health issues or consequences resulting from the use or misuse of the information contained in this book. Individual results may vary, and the suggestions herein may not be suitable for everyone. Readers are encouraged to consult with healthcare professionals before making any changes to their diet, exercise, or lifestyle routines.

ELITE

NUTRITION RESEARCH

Elite Nutrition Research is a science-driven health and education company dedicated to understanding and optimizing human physiology at its most fundamental level. Our work is built on an architecture-first approach—examining how nutrients interact with cellular systems, membranes, energy production, and signaling pathways to shape overall health and performance. Rather than following trends, we focus on first principles, combining biochemical insight, formulation precision, and practical application to create both advanced nutritional products and in-depth educational systems.

Through our books, courses, and formulations, Elite Nutrition Research aims to give individuals direct access to the mechanisms that govern their biology empowering them to think clearly, act intentionally, and build lasting health from the inside out.

To explore our full system of products, courses, and research, visit:
www.elitenutritionresearch.com

Table of Contents

PART I

THE COLLAPSE OF THINKING

Chapter 1

Breakdown of Feedback and Reality Alignment

A functional thinking system depends on continuous exposure to reality. It generates a model, acts on that model, receives an outcome, and then compares the result against the prediction. The difference between the two is not incidental. It is the mechanism that drives correction. When the gap is detected, the system adjusts its internal structure so that future predictions better match external conditions. This loop is what keeps perception aligned. It is not optional. Without it, thinking becomes detached from the environment it is supposed to represent.

The integrity of this loop depends on the quality of feedback. Feedback must be immediate enough to connect cause and effect, clear enough to distinguish signal from noise, and consistent enough to allow patterns to be recognized. When these conditions are met, the system refines itself automatically. Errors cannot persist because they are exposed. Incorrect assumptions collapse under repeated contradiction. Accurate models stabilize because they continue to produce reliable results. Over time, this produces a system that converges toward reality through repeated correction.

When feedback weakens, this process begins to fail at the structural level. The system still produces predictions and still takes action, but the outcome no longer provides a clean signal. Time delays separate decision from consequence. Intervening variables obscure the relationship between input and result. Multiple actions overlap before prior outcomes are resolved. Under these conditions, the system loses its ability to isolate cause and effect. It cannot determine which part of the model produced the outcome, so it cannot update that model with precision.

Modern environments amplify this breakdown. Decisions are routed through layers of abstraction that buffer their consequences. Financial systems distribute risk across time and participants. Social systems reinforce beliefs independent of accuracy. Technological systems automate execution without requiring understanding. Each layer increases the distance between action and outcome. The system continues to operate, but the connection between what it does and what happens becomes progressively less visible. Without that visibility, correction becomes inconsistent.

Delay is the primary disruptor. When an outcome arrives long after the decision that caused it, the system struggles to associate the two. The internal model remains unchanged because the feedback signal arrives outside the window where it can be integrated. By the time the consequence is observed, the system has already moved on, producing new decisions based on the same flawed structure. This creates accumulation. Errors are repeated because they are not identified at the point where correction would be effective.

Distortion compounds the problem. Feedback is rarely received in a neutral form. It is filtered through interpretation, social context, and prior beliefs. A negative outcome may be attributed to external factors rather than internal error. A positive outcome may reinforce a flawed model if the success occurred by coincidence rather than accuracy. The system begins to evaluate itself based on perceived outcomes rather than actual causal relationships. This introduces noise into the correction process. Adjustments are made, but they are not aligned with the underlying structure of reality.

In the absence of reliable feedback, the system shifts its reference point inward. Instead of comparing predictions to outcomes, it compares outputs to internal states. Coherence becomes a substitute for correctness. If a conclusion feels consistent with prior beliefs or aligns with an existing narrative, it is accepted. This reduces cognitive load because it removes the need for external validation, but it also removes the constraint that keeps the system grounded. The model becomes self-reinforcing. It evolves based on internal agreement rather than external accuracy.

This transition changes how error behaves. In a feedback-driven system, error is localized and correctable. It appears as a mismatch between expectation and result, and it can be traced back to a specific assumption or relationship within the model. In a feedback-degraded system, error becomes distributed. It is embedded across multiple assumptions, each of which appears internally consistent. Because the system lacks a clear signal indicating where the failure occurred, it cannot isolate the source. Corrections, when attempted, tend to address surface-level outputs rather than the structure that produced them.

Over time, the model drifts. The system continues to operate, but its representation of reality becomes less accurate with each cycle. Decisions still produce outcomes, but those outcomes are no longer predictable. Variability increases. The same input produces different results depending on context, timing, and interacting variables that are not properly accounted for. This unpredictability is not randomness. It is the result of a model that no longer reflects the structure of the environment it is navigating.

The breakdown of feedback does not produce immediate failure. It produces a gradual loss of alignment. Early in the process, the system compensates. It adjusts behavior heuristically, relying on shortcuts and approximations to maintain function. These adjustments can sustain performance temporarily, especially in environments that tolerate error. But they do not restore structural accuracy. They allow the system to operate while the underlying model continues to degrade.

Eventually, the accumulation reaches a threshold where compensation is no longer sufficient. Outcomes begin to diverge consistently from expectations. Decisions that once produced acceptable results now fail more frequently. The system experiences this as instability, but the instability is not new. It has been developing over time as feedback weakened and corrections stopped occurring at the structural level.

What appears as sudden failure is the visible expression of long-standing misalignment.

Restoring alignment requires reestablishing the feedback loop. The system must reduce delay, remove distortion, and reconnect decisions to their outcomes in a way that allows cause and effect to be observed directly. This does not require more information. It requires cleaner signals. When the system can once again compare prediction to result with clarity, correction resumes. Models begin to update. Accuracy increases incrementally with each cycle. The process is mechanical. When feedback is restored, alignment follows.

The Death of Clear Thought

Clear thought does not disappear because the brain loses capacity. It disappears when the system that enforces correction stops functioning. A thinking system remains accurate only when it is continuously exposed to consequences that are tightly linked to its decisions. Action produces an outcome, the outcome is compared to the expectation, and the model is adjusted based on the difference. This sequence maintains alignment because error cannot remain hidden. When the link between decision and consequence is immediate and visible, inaccurate thinking is unstable. It is forced to change or it produces results that cannot be sustained.

In environments where consequence is delayed or absorbed, this pressure is removed. The system continues to generate decisions, but those decisions are no longer evaluated against a clear signal. The outcome still occurs, but it is separated from the action that produced it by time, complexity, or intermediaries. Without a direct connection, the system cannot reliably assign cause. It observes results, but it cannot determine which part of its internal model led to them. This breaks the correction mechanism. The model persists not because it is accurate, but because it is not being challenged in a way the system can process.

Immediate consequence serves as a constraint. It limits the range of viable models by eliminating those that do not match reality. When that constraint weakens, the system gains the ability to operate under inaccurate assumptions without immediate failure. This creates a shift in behavior. Instead of refining models to match external structure, the system begins to optimize for internal coherence and short-term output. It selects conclusions that feel consistent, that resolve quickly, or that align with prior beliefs, because there is no strong external signal forcing it to do otherwise.

Weakened feedback loops introduce ambiguity into every stage of reasoning. The system still forms expectations, but it cannot verify them with precision. It still observes outcomes, but those outcomes arrive without clear attribution. Multiple variables interact before the result is visible, making it difficult to isolate which factor mattered. The system responds by reducing the depth of analysis required to reach a conclusion. It relies more heavily on compressed representations of reality, because those require less processing and can function in the absence of clear validation.

This shift does not produce an immediate collapse. It produces drift. The model begins to move away from reality in small increments, each one uncorrected because the feedback signal is too weak or too delayed to trigger adjustment. Early errors remain embedded in the structure, influencing future decisions. As new inputs are processed through this distorted model, additional error is introduced. The system continues to operate, but its outputs become less predictable because they are no longer anchored to stable relationships.

At the same time, reinforcement begins to come from the wrong source. Instead of being validated by outcomes, conclusions are reinforced by repetition, agreement, or emotional alignment. A belief that is shared or frequently repeated begins to feel correct regardless of its correspondence to reality. This creates a secondary feedback loop that operates entirely within the system. It strengthens internal patterns without reference to external conditions. Over time, this loop can dominate, making the system resistant to correction even when contradictory evidence becomes available.

The absence of immediate consequence also changes how error is experienced. When correction is delayed, the system does not register the cost of a flawed decision at the point where it could adjust its model. The consequence appears later, often disconnected from the original cause. By then, the system has already made additional decisions based on the same flawed structure. The cost accumulates, but it is not attributed correctly. This prevents targeted correction. The system may attempt to change behavior, but without identifying the structural source of error, those changes remain superficial.

As this process continues, clear thought is replaced by functional output. The system is still active. It still produces conclusions, makes decisions, and navigates its environment. But the underlying mechanism that ensures those outputs align with reality has degraded. Thinking becomes a process of generating answers rather than validating them. The distinction is subtle at first, but it defines the trajectory of the system. One path leads toward increasing accuracy through correction. The other leads toward increasing divergence sustained by internal reinforcement.

Restoring clear thought requires reestablishing consequence as a usable signal. The system must once again experience outcomes in a way that allows cause and effect to be linked directly. This reduces ambiguity and forces the model to confront discrepancies between expectation and result. When the feedback loop is restored to sufficient strength, inaccurate structures become unstable again. They are exposed, adjusted, and replaced. Clear thinking does not need to be imposed. It re-emerges when the conditions that enforce alignment are present.

Delayed Consequences and Model Drift

A thinking system depends on temporal proximity between action and consequence. When a decision produces an outcome within a narrow time window, the system can bind the two together. The model that generated the decision is evaluated against the result, and any mismatch can be traced back to a specific assumption or relationship within that model. This binding process is what allows correction to occur with precision. It is not enough for consequences to exist. They must arrive while the system still retains a clear representation of the decision that produced them.

As the delay between action and outcome increases, this binding begins to fail. The system moves forward, generating new decisions and processing new inputs before the consequence of the previous decision becomes visible. By the time the outcome appears, the internal state that produced the original action has already shifted. Variables have changed. Context has evolved. The system is no longer operating under the same conditions. This breaks continuity. The outcome cannot be cleanly attached to the decision, and without that attachment, the model cannot be updated accurately.

This introduces ambiguity into causation. When a result emerges after multiple intervening steps, the system is forced to infer which variables contributed to it. It cannot directly observe the relationship. It reconstructs it. This reconstruction relies on incomplete information and is influenced by the system's existing biases and assumptions. Instead of isolating the true cause, it often attributes the outcome to the most visible or recent factor. This creates misalignment at the structural level. The system adjusts the wrong part of its model, leaving the actual source of error intact.

Model drift begins as a consequence of this misattribution. Each time an outcome is incorrectly linked to its cause, the internal structure shifts in a direction that does not correspond to reality. The system believes it has corrected itself, but the correction is misapplied. Over repeated cycles, these small deviations accumulate. The model becomes progressively less accurate, not because it is static, but because it is updating in the wrong direction. Adaptation continues, but it no longer improves alignment.

Time delays also reduce the perceived cost of error. When consequences are immediate, the system experiences the full impact of a flawed decision at the point where the decision can still be associated with its cause. This creates a strong signal that drives correction. When consequences are delayed, that signal weakens. The system does not feel the cost when the decision is made. It experiences the outcome later, often in a different context where the connection is less apparent. This disconnect reduces the urgency of correction. Errors are tolerated longer because their effects are not directly linked to their origin.

As delays increase further, the system begins to operate on overlapping decision cycles. Multiple actions are taken before any of their outcomes are fully realized. When results begin to appear, they represent the combined effects of several prior decisions rather than a single identifiable cause. The system is now evaluating composite outcomes. It sees the result, but it cannot decompose it into its contributing parts with sufficient resolution. This prevents targeted adjustment. Changes to the model become broad and imprecise, affecting multiple variables without isolating which one actually mattered.

This environment favors simplified reasoning strategies. Instead of attempting to track complex, delayed relationships, the system compresses its model. It reduces the number of variables it actively considers and relies on surface-level patterns to guide decisions. These strategies are efficient under conditions of uncertainty, but they sacrifice accuracy. They allow the system to continue operating despite the breakdown in feedback, but they do not restore alignment. They stabilize output at the cost of precision.

Drift becomes visible when predictions consistently fail to match outcomes, but even then the system may struggle to identify why. The internal model remains coherent. Each adjustment made along the way appeared justified based on the information available at the time. The divergence is not experienced as a single error, but as a gradual shift that never triggered a strong enough signal to force correction. By the time the misalignment is obvious, it is distributed across many interconnected assumptions, making it difficult to reverse.

The separation of decision and outcome does not remove causality. It obscures it. The underlying relationships remain intact, but the system loses access to them in a usable form. Restoring alignment requires reducing this separation. Shortening feedback loops, isolating variables, and observing outcomes in closer proximity to decisions allows the system to rebuild accurate cause-and-effect mapping. When temporal distance is reduced, binding returns. The system can once again attach outcomes to the decisions that produced them, and model correction resumes with clarity.

The Collapse of Self-Correction

A thinking system maintains accuracy only if it can revise its internal structure when outcomes contradict its expectations. This requires more than detecting error. It requires the ability to trace that error back to a specific component of the model and modify it without destabilizing the rest of the system. Self-correction is therefore a structural property. It depends on how tightly predictions are linked to outcomes, how clearly causes can be isolated, and how safely the system can update itself without losing coherence. When these conditions hold, incorrect models are inherently unstable. They are exposed through mismatch and replaced through adjustment.

The collapse begins when mismatch is no longer treated as a signal that demands structural change. This can occur when outcomes are ambiguous, delayed, or filtered through interpretation before they are evaluated. The system still detects that something is off, but the signal is weak or unclear. Without a precise mapping between prediction and result, the system cannot identify which part of the model produced the error. It registers discrepancy without localization. Under these conditions, updating becomes risky. Any change could disrupt parts of the model that are still functioning, so the system defaults to preserving its existing structure.

To maintain stability in the absence of clear correction signals, the system shifts toward protecting coherence rather than improving accuracy. Internal consistency becomes the primary constraint. A model that explains itself without contradiction is favored over one that aligns with external outcomes but requires structural revision. This shift is subtle but decisive. The system continues to process information, but it evaluates new inputs based on how well they fit the existing model rather than whether they improve its correspondence to reality. Inputs that align are integrated. Inputs that conflict are reinterpreted, minimized, or excluded.

This process introduces a form of structural inertia. Once a model reaches a certain level of internal coherence, it becomes resistant to change even when it produces incorrect predictions. Error no longer triggers revision. It triggers reinterpretation. The system adjusts the narrative around the outcome instead of adjusting the mechanism that generated the prediction. This preserves stability in the short term, but it allows misalignment to persist and accumulate. Over time, the model becomes increasingly detached from the structure it is meant to represent.

Energy and complexity also play a role. Updating a model requires computational effort. It involves re-evaluating relationships, integrating new information, and potentially restructuring large portions of the system. When feedback is unclear, the expected benefit of this effort decreases. The system cannot reliably determine whether a change will improve accuracy, so it reduces the frequency of updates. It shifts toward lower-cost strategies such as reinforcing existing patterns or applying local adjustments that do not require full structural revision. These strategies conserve resources, but they do not correct underlying errors.

As updates become less frequent and less precise, the system begins to operate on increasingly outdated representations. It continues to generate predictions, but those predictions are based on assumptions that have not been tested or refined against recent outcomes. This creates a widening gap between the model and the environment. The system may still function in stable conditions where the environment does not change significantly, but its ability to adapt declines. When conditions shift, the model lacks the flexibility to adjust because the mechanisms responsible for updating have degraded.

Another factor is the loss of traceability within the reasoning process. In a system that can self-correct effectively, the path from input to conclusion is structured and inspectable. Each step can be examined, allowing errors to be located and corrected at their source. When reasoning becomes compressed or associative, this path is no longer clear. The system arrives at conclusions without maintaining a detailed record of how it got there. When an output is incorrect, there is no defined point within the process where the error can be isolated. Without traceability, correction becomes guesswork. The system may change outputs, but it cannot reliably fix the mechanism that produced them.

Over time, these factors converge. Weak feedback reduces the clarity of error signals. Structural inertia discourages revision. Energy constraints favor low-cost strategies. Loss of traceability prevents precise correction. The system reaches a state where it continues to operate despite being misaligned, but it no longer has a functional pathway to restore accuracy. It can detect that outcomes are not matching expectations, but it cannot translate that detection into effective structural change.

The result is a stable but inaccurate system. It maintains internal consistency, generates continuous output, and resists disruption, but its predictions do not reliably correspond to reality. Because the system still functions, the failure is not immediately obvious. It appears as gradual degradation in performance rather than a clear breakdown. By the time the misalignment becomes visible, it is embedded across multiple layers of the model, making correction difficult and resource-intensive.

Restoring self-correction requires reestablishing the conditions that make updating both possible and necessary. The system must regain access to clear, localized feedback signals that allow errors to be traced to their source. It must reduce the cost of revision by structuring models in a way that allows components to be updated without destabilizing the whole. It must reintroduce traceability so that the path from input to output can be examined and adjusted. When these conditions are restored, incorrect models lose their stability. They are exposed through mismatch and replaced through targeted correction, and the system regains its ability to align itself with the structure it is attempting to represent.

Chapter 2

Speed Over Accuracy

A thinking system always operates under constraints. It has limited time, limited processing capacity, and a continuous stream of inputs that demand response. Under stable conditions with clear feedback, the system can allocate resources toward accuracy. It can slow down, evaluate relationships in detail, and refine its internal model through repeated comparison with outcomes. When the environment changes to favor rapid response, this allocation shifts. Speed becomes the dominant constraint, and the system reorganizes itself to produce outputs quickly rather than precisely. This is not a conscious choice. It is a structural adaptation to the conditions under which the system is operating.

The shift toward speed changes how information is processed at every stage. Instead of constructing a detailed representation of the problem, the system compresses it. It reduces the number of variables it actively tracks and prioritizes those that are most immediately visible or most easily processed. Relationships that require extended analysis are ignored or approximated. This allows the system to generate a conclusion with less computational effort, but it also removes the depth required to maintain accuracy. The output is faster because the process that produces it has been simplified.

This simplification alters the structure of reasoning itself. In a system optimized for accuracy, conclusions are built through sequential evaluation. Inputs are examined, relationships are tested, and intermediate steps are validated before the final output is produced.

Each stage acts as a checkpoint, ensuring that errors are identified and corrected before they propagate. When speed becomes the priority, these checkpoints are reduced or eliminated. The system moves from input to conclusion through a shorter pathway, often bypassing intermediate validation. This increases throughput, but it also increases the probability that errors will pass through the system undetected.

To sustain this mode of operation, the system relies on pattern compression. Instead of analyzing each situation from first principles, it maps current inputs onto previously encountered patterns and retrieves a corresponding response. This is efficient because it replaces computation with recall. The system does not need to evaluate every variable if it can recognize the situation as similar to one it has seen before. However, this approach depends on the accuracy of the stored patterns and the degree to which the current situation actually matches them. When the match is incomplete or misleading, the system applies an inappropriate response with high confidence.

Speed also changes how uncertainty is handled. In an accuracy-driven system, uncertainty triggers further analysis. The system expands its model, gathers additional information, and delays the decision until confidence reaches an acceptable level. In a speed-driven system, uncertainty is compressed or ignored. The system resolves ambiguity by selecting the most accessible interpretation and proceeding as if it were sufficient. This allows the decision to be completed quickly, but it reduces the reliability of the outcome because the underlying uncertainty has not been addressed.

The environment reinforces this behavior. Rapid feedback cycles reward quick responses even when they are only partially correct. Delayed consequences obscure the cost of inaccuracy, while immediate rewards reinforce the act of producing an answer. Over time, the system learns that generating output quickly is more valuable than ensuring that output is correct. This learning is not abstract. It is encoded in the structure of the system. Pathways that produce rapid conclusions are strengthened through repeated use, while pathways that require deeper analysis are used less frequently and become less accessible.

As this process continues, the system develops a bias toward completion. The goal shifts from producing an accurate model to producing a finished answer. Once an output is generated, the system moves on to the next input rather than revisiting the decision to evaluate its correctness. This reduces the opportunity for post-decision correction. Errors that might have been identified through reflection remain embedded in the model because the system does not allocate resources to re-examining them.

The cumulative effect is a reduction in precision. Individual errors may appear minor, but they are not isolated. Each output becomes an input for future decisions. When those outputs are based on compressed or incomplete representations, the errors propagate forward. The system continues to operate at high speed, but its internal model becomes less accurate with each cycle. This creates a divergence between perceived understanding and actual alignment with reality.

The shift toward speed does not eliminate the system's ability to reason. It changes the conditions under which reasoning occurs. The system remains capable of detailed analysis, but it does not engage that capability unless the environment demands it. In the absence of strong feedback or explicit constraints, it defaults to the faster mode because it is more efficient. This makes accuracy situational rather than consistent. The system can produce correct results, but it does not do so reliably across different contexts.

Restoring accuracy requires changing the constraints under which the system operates. Time must be reintroduced as a resource that can be allocated toward analysis. Decisions must be evaluated against outcomes in a way that makes errors visible and costly. The system must be forced to maintain intermediate steps in its reasoning process so that those steps can be inspected and corrected. When these conditions are present, the pathways that support accurate reasoning become active again. Speed remains available, but it no longer dominates the structure of the system. Accuracy becomes stable because it is supported by the architecture rather than dependent on intermittent effort.

The Speed Trap

A thinking system can increase output by reducing the amount of processing applied to each input. This is the core tradeoff between throughput and precision. When more decisions are required within a fixed time window, the system compresses its evaluation process so that it can complete more cycles. Each individual decision receives less scrutiny, fewer variables are considered, and intermediate validation steps are removed. The system appears more productive because it produces a higher volume of outputs, but the structure that ensures those outputs are accurate has been reduced.

Precision depends on depth. A precise decision requires the system to construct a representation of the problem that includes relevant variables, test relationships between them, and verify that the conclusion follows from those relationships. This takes time and computational effort. When throughput becomes the priority, the system cannot sustain this level of processing for every input. It begins to approximate. It selects a subset of variables that are easiest to access, assumes relationships rather than testing them, and moves directly to a conclusion. The output is generated quickly, but it is based on an incomplete model.

As this pattern repeats, the internal architecture adapts. Pathways that support rapid completion are reinforced because they are used more frequently. Pathways that support deeper analysis are used less often and become less accessible. The system does not lose the ability to reason with precision, but it loses the tendency to do so. Precision becomes optional rather than default. In most cases, the system selects the faster pathway because it satisfies the immediate demand for output.

This shift introduces systematic error. Each decision made with reduced precision carries a higher probability of being incorrect or partially correct. These errors are not isolated events. They become inputs for subsequent decisions. The system builds on its own outputs, so inaccuracies propagate forward through the model. Over time, the accumulation of small errors alters the structure of the system's understanding. The model begins to reflect the approximations used to generate outputs rather than the relationships present in the environment.

Throughput also changes how the system evaluates success. When output volume is high, completion itself becomes a metric. The system receives reinforcement for finishing decisions quickly, independent of their accuracy. This reinforcement strengthens the pathways that produce rapid outputs and further reduces the use of slower, more precise processes. The system learns that speed satisfies the constraint, while accuracy is not consistently measured. As a result, it allocates resources toward maximizing throughput rather than maintaining alignment with reality.

The loss of precision reduces traceability within the reasoning process. When a decision is produced through a compressed pathway, the intermediate steps are either absent or not explicitly represented. The system arrives at a conclusion without maintaining a clear record of how it was derived. When the output is incorrect, there is no defined location within the process where the error can be isolated. Correction becomes difficult because the structure that would allow the system to inspect and adjust its reasoning is no longer present.

In this state, the system becomes dependent on external correction. It cannot reliably detect its own errors because it lacks the internal structure required to evaluate them. If feedback is strong and immediate, this dependence can be partially offset. Errors are identified externally and the system adjusts its outputs accordingly. If feedback is weak or delayed, errors persist. The system continues to produce high volumes of output, but the alignment between those outputs and reality degrades.

The speed trap is not simply an increase in pace. It is a reconfiguration of the system's architecture. By prioritizing throughput, the system removes the mechanisms that maintain precision. It trades depth for volume, validation for completion, and traceability for efficiency. This tradeoff is not inherently harmful if it is applied selectively, but when it becomes the default mode of operation, it alters the system's ability to maintain accuracy over time.

Escaping the speed trap requires restoring the structural elements that support precision. The system must reintroduce intermediate validation steps so that conclusions are built rather than retrieved. It must maintain explicit representations of how decisions are derived so that errors can be traced and corrected. It must evaluate outputs based on their correspondence to outcomes rather than the speed at which they are produced. When these elements are present, throughput can be increased without collapsing precision, because the architecture that enforces accuracy remains intact.

Heuristic Substitution

A thinking system reduces computational load by substituting full evaluation with compressed decision rules. Instead of constructing a detailed model for each problem, it maps the current input onto a stored pattern and retrieves a response associated with that pattern. This substitution replaces a sequence of explicit steps with a direct transition from input to output. The process is efficient because it minimizes the number of variables that must be actively processed. It allows the system to operate under time constraints and high input volume without exceeding its capacity.

Pattern recognition depends on similarity. The system must determine whether the current input matches a previously encountered configuration closely enough to justify using the same response. When the match is accurate, this produces acceptable results with minimal effort. The system avoids recomputing relationships that have already been established. However, the decision to treat two situations as equivalent is itself a critical step. If the system compresses this step, it may accept a partial match as sufficient. This introduces error at the point of substitution. The response is applied not because the underlying structure is the same, but because the surface features appear similar.

Structured reasoning operates differently. It decomposes the problem into components, evaluates relationships between those components, and constructs a conclusion that follows from those relationships. Each step is explicit. Variables are defined, interactions are tested, and assumptions can be inspected. This allows the system to adjust individual parts of the process when an error is detected. Precision is maintained because the pathway from input to output is transparent and can be modified at specific points.

When heuristic substitution becomes the dominant mode, this structure is reduced. The system no longer maintains a detailed pathway. It relies on the stored association between pattern and response, and that association may not encode the full set of relationships present in the original situation. Over time, the system accumulates a library of compressed mappings that allow it to respond quickly, but these mappings are approximations. They capture regularities in the environment without preserving the underlying structure that produced those regularities.

This shift alters how error propagates. In a structured system, an incorrect conclusion can be traced back to a specific step where an assumption or calculation failed. The system can isolate that step and modify it without affecting unrelated parts of the model. In a heuristic-driven system, the error is embedded in the mapping itself. The pattern-response pair does not expose its internal logic, so the system cannot identify which aspect of the mapping is incorrect. Correction requires replacing or adjusting the entire mapping, often without clear guidance on what should change.

Heuristic substitution also changes how new information is integrated. When the system encounters data that does not fit an existing pattern, it can either expand its pattern library or attempt to force the input into a known category. Under time pressure, the latter is more likely. The system selects the closest available match and proceeds, even if the fit is incomplete. This preserves speed, but it prevents the model from incorporating new structure. Inputs that could refine the system are instead absorbed into existing patterns, reinforcing their use without improving their accuracy.

As reliance on heuristics increases, the system becomes more sensitive to surface features and less responsive to underlying relationships. It prioritizes what is immediately recognizable over what is structurally relevant. This can produce consistent outputs in familiar environments where patterns are stable, but it reduces adaptability. When conditions change or when inputs differ in ways that are not captured by existing patterns, the system applies responses that are no longer appropriate. Because the process is compressed, it does not detect the mismatch before producing the output.

The substitution of heuristics for structured reasoning does not eliminate reasoning capacity. It reallocates it. The system retains the ability to perform detailed analysis, but it engages that capability less frequently because the heuristic pathway satisfies most immediate demands. Over time, this reduces the system's tendency to construct explicit models. It defaults to retrieval rather than evaluation, even in situations where a full analysis would be required to maintain accuracy.

Restoring structured reasoning requires reintroducing the steps that heuristics bypass. The system must explicitly define variables, test relationships, and construct conclusions through intermediate stages that can be inspected. This increases computational cost per decision, but it restores traceability and precision. Heuristics can still be used where patterns are well-established and the cost of error is low, but they must remain subordinate to a structure that can evaluate and correct them. When that structure is active, pattern recognition becomes a tool within the system rather than the mechanism that defines it.

Emotional Coherence as False Truth

A thinking system requires an external reference to maintain accuracy. Predictions must be compared to outcomes, and conclusions must be constrained by conditions that exist outside the system itself. This external alignment prevents the model from drifting. It limits which interpretations can persist because only those that correspond to reality continue to produce stable results. When this reference weakens, the system does not stop producing conclusions. It replaces the external constraint with an internal one. Coherence becomes the primary filter. If a conclusion fits within the existing structure of beliefs and produces a stable internal state, it is accepted as valid.

Emotional coherence provides a low-cost mechanism for maintaining this internal consistency. When a conclusion aligns with prior beliefs, reduces internal conflict, or produces a sense of resolution, it is processed as correct. This response is immediate and does not require validation against external outcomes. The system can resolve uncertainty quickly by selecting interpretations that maintain internal stability. This reduces computational demand and allows rapid output, but it removes the requirement that conclusions correspond to actual conditions. The model begins to optimize for internal equilibrium rather than external accuracy.

This substitution changes how information is evaluated. Inputs are no longer assessed based on whether they improve the model's ability to predict outcomes. They are assessed based on how they interact with the existing structure. Information that reinforces current patterns is integrated easily. It strengthens the internal network because it increases consistency across components. Information that conflicts with the model creates instability. It introduces discrepancies that would require structural revision to resolve. Under conditions where feedback is weak and speed is prioritized, the system avoids this cost by modifying the interpretation of the input rather than the structure of the model.

As this process continues, the system develops a closed loop. Conclusions reinforce beliefs, beliefs shape interpretation, and interpretation determines which inputs are accepted or rejected. This loop operates independently of external validation. It maintains coherence internally even as alignment with reality degrades. The system experiences this as clarity because contradictions are minimized within the model. However, this clarity is not derived from accurate mapping. It is the result of filtering out information that would expose misalignment.

Internal consistency is not inherently inaccurate. A model can be both internally coherent and externally aligned. The problem arises when coherence is used as a substitute for alignment rather than as a complement to it. When the system treats the absence of internal contradiction as sufficient evidence of correctness, it removes the need to test its assumptions against outcomes. This allows structurally flawed models to persist as long as they remain self-consistent.

The reliance on emotional coherence also affects how error is processed. In a feedback-driven system, error produces a discrepancy that must be resolved through structural change. In a coherence-driven system, error produces discomfort that must be resolved through interpretation. The system reduces this discomfort by adjusting the narrative around the outcome. It attributes failure to external factors, reframes the result as an exception, or selectively focuses on aspects of the outcome that appear consistent with the model. These adjustments preserve internal stability, but they prevent the model from updating in a way that would improve accuracy.

Over time, the model becomes insulated from correction. It no longer requires agreement with external conditions to remain stable. It only requires internal consistency. This insulation allows increasingly large discrepancies to accumulate without triggering structural revision. The system continues to function because it can generate coherent explanations for its outputs, but those explanations are not constrained by reality. They are constructed to maintain internal alignment rather than to reflect external structure.

This shift reduces adaptability. When conditions change, a system aligned with external feedback adjusts because its model is continuously updated based on outcomes. A system aligned with internal coherence resists change because new information that contradicts the model is filtered or reinterpreted. The system maintains stability in the short term, but it loses the ability to respond effectively to new conditions. It operates on a representation that no longer matches the environment, and its decisions reflect that misalignment.

Restoring external alignment requires reestablishing outcome-based validation as the primary constraint. Conclusions must be tested against results rather than accepted based on how they feel within the model. The system must allow internal instability to occur when discrepancies are detected, because that instability is the signal that drives correction. Emotional coherence can support function by maintaining continuity, but it cannot define truth. When external feedback is reintroduced as the governing reference, internally consistent but inaccurate models lose their stability, and the system regains its capacity to update based on the structure it is interacting with.

Chapter 3

Unstructured Cognition

A thinking system produces reliable outputs only when its internal processes are organized into defined stages that preserve relationships between inputs, transformations, and conclusions. Structure provides continuity. It ensures that each step in the process is connected to the one before it and constrained by the one after it. Inputs are translated into representations, those representations are evaluated through explicit relationships, and conclusions emerge from that sequence. When this structure is intact, reasoning remains stable because each output can be traced back through the pathway that produced it. Error can be located, and the system can adjust the specific component responsible without disrupting the entire model.

Unstructured cognition emerges when this pathway is no longer maintained. The system continues to process inputs and generate outputs, but the intermediate steps are compressed or omitted. Instead of moving through defined stages, the system transitions directly from stimulus to conclusion through associative links that are not explicitly represented. These links are formed through repeated exposure and reinforced by prior use, allowing rapid response without reconstructing the full chain of reasoning. The system appears to function normally because it continues to produce answers, but the underlying process that ensures those answers correspond to reality has degraded.

This change alters how information is handled at the point of entry. In a structured system, inputs are parsed into components that can be individually evaluated. Variables are identified, relationships are mapped, and irrelevant data is filtered based on defined criteria. In an unstructured system, inputs are processed as wholes. The system responds to the overall pattern rather than decomposing it into parts. This reduces processing time, but it removes the ability to isolate which elements of the input are actually driving the response. The output reflects the general impression of the input rather than a constructed understanding of it.

As processing continues, the absence of structure prevents the system from maintaining consistent relationships between variables. In a structured pathway, relationships are explicitly defined and tested. The system can determine how a change in one variable affects another and adjust its model accordingly. In an unstructured pathway, these relationships are implicit. They are embedded within associative patterns that do not expose their internal logic. When conditions change, the system cannot adjust specific relationships because it does not represent them explicitly. It can only modify the overall pattern, often without understanding which component required adjustment.

This lack of explicit representation removes traceability. When an output is incorrect, the system cannot reconstruct the sequence of steps that led to it because that sequence was never fully formed. The conclusion exists, but the pathway that produced it is not accessible. Without traceability, correction becomes diffuse. The system may change future outputs based on new inputs, but it cannot target the structural source of the error. This leads to inconsistent adjustments that do not reliably improve accuracy.

Unstructured cognition also increases sensitivity to context. Because the system relies on associative links rather than defined relationships, small changes in input can produce large changes in output. The same underlying problem may generate different conclusions depending on how it is presented, because the system is responding to surface features rather than stable structures. This variability reduces predictability. The system cannot guarantee consistent outputs because it does not operate on a consistent internal framework.

The shift toward unstructured processing is reinforced by environments that prioritize speed and volume. When inputs arrive continuously and decisions must be made quickly, the system favors pathways that minimize processing time. Associative links provide a direct route from input to output, allowing rapid response without constructing a full model. Over time, repeated use of these pathways strengthens them, while structured processes that require more effort are used less frequently. The system adapts by making unstructured cognition its default mode.

As this adaptation progresses, the system loses the ability to scale its reasoning. Structured cognition allows complexity to be managed because it breaks problems into components that can be analyzed independently and then recombined. Unstructured cognition does not support this decomposition. As problems increase in complexity, the system cannot maintain a coherent representation of all relevant variables. It relies on partial patterns that capture only a subset of the problem, leading to outputs that are incomplete or inaccurate.

The degradation is not immediately obvious because the system remains functional in simple or familiar contexts. Associative processing can produce acceptable results when patterns are stable and well-established. The limitations become visible when the system encounters novel situations or problems that require precise relationships to be understood. In these cases, the lack of structure prevents accurate modeling, and the system's outputs diverge from reality.

Restoring structured cognition requires rebuilding the pathway from input to output. Inputs must be decomposed into variables that can be explicitly represented. Relationships between those variables must be defined and tested. Intermediate steps must be maintained so that conclusions are constructed rather than retrieved. This increases processing cost, but it restores traceability and allows errors to be corrected at their source. When structure is reestablished, the system regains its ability to produce consistent, accurate outputs across varying conditions because its reasoning is once again anchored in defined relationships rather than associative shortcuts.

Thinking Without Structure

A structured thinking system constructs conclusions through defined relationships between variables. It identifies components within an input, establishes how those components interact, and moves step by step toward an output that follows from those interactions. Each stage in the process is constrained by the previous one. This creates continuity. The conclusion is not simply reached. It is built. Because the pathway is explicit, the system can examine each step, verify its validity, and adjust specific elements when errors occur.

When structure degrades, this pathway is replaced by association chains. Instead of evaluating relationships directly, the system moves from one concept to another based on proximity, familiarity, or prior co-occurrence. The transition between steps is not governed by defined rules. It is governed by linkage strength. Inputs activate related patterns, those patterns activate additional patterns, and the system follows this chain until it arrives at a conclusion. The output emerges from the sequence, but the sequence itself does not represent a tested set of relationships. It represents a path through stored associations.

Association chains reduce the need for explicit computation. The system does not need to construct a model of the problem if it can traverse a pathway that has been reinforced through prior use. This allows rapid response, especially in environments where time is limited. However, the efficiency comes from bypassing evaluation. The system does not test whether each transition in the chain is valid in the current context. It assumes validity based on prior linkage. When the context differs from the conditions under which the chain was formed, this assumption introduces error.

Inference operates under a different constraint. It requires that each step in the reasoning process maintain a defined relationship to the input. The system must ensure that transitions between steps are justified by the structure of the problem rather than by the strength of association. This maintains alignment because the conclusion is anchored to the relationships present in the input. When inference is replaced by association, this constraint is removed. The system can arrive at a conclusion that feels connected to the input without being derived from it.

This shift alters how consistency is maintained. In a structured system, consistency arises from the coherence of relationships. Each part of the model fits because it has been constructed through compatible interactions between variables. In an association-driven system, consistency arises from the continuity of the chain. As long as each step leads smoothly to the next, the sequence feels coherent. The system does not require that the chain accurately represent the underlying structure of the problem. It only requires that the transitions are not disruptive.

The loss of structure also removes checkpoints. Inference includes implicit validation at each stage because relationships are examined before the system proceeds. If a step does not hold, the process stops or adjusts. Association chains do not include these checkpoints. The system progresses through the chain without pausing to evaluate whether each transition is valid. This allows uninterrupted flow, but it also allows invalid steps to pass through the process and influence the final output.

Error within association chains is difficult to isolate. When a conclusion is incorrect, the system cannot easily identify which link in the chain introduced the error. Each transition appears locally coherent because it is based on an existing association. The chain as a whole may be misaligned, but the system lacks a representation of the relationships that would allow it to evaluate each step independently. Correction becomes imprecise. The system may avoid similar chains in the future or adjust surface-level outputs, but it cannot reliably modify the specific transition that caused the failure.

As reliance on association increases, the system becomes more sensitive to initial conditions. The starting point of the chain determines the path that follows. Small differences in input can activate different associations, leading to divergent outputs even when the underlying problem is similar. This reduces stability. The system cannot guarantee consistent reasoning because it does not operate on a fixed structure. It operates on pathways that are contingent on activation patterns.

The replacement of inference with association does not eliminate the system's ability to reason structurally. It reduces the frequency with which that ability is used. The system defaults to association because it satisfies immediate demands for speed and efficiency. Over time, the pathways that support inference are used less often, and the system becomes less likely to engage them even when the situation requires it. Structured reasoning becomes available but inactive.

Reestablishing inference requires interrupting the association chain and rebuilding the pathway step by step. The system must identify variables explicitly, define the relationships between them, and ensure that each transition in the reasoning process is justified by those relationships. This introduces friction. It slows the process and increases computational demand. However, it restores alignment because the conclusion is once again derived from the structure of the problem rather than from the sequence of associations. When inference is active, association can still operate as a preliminary filter, but it no longer determines the outcome.

Narrative Over Logic

A structured thinking system evaluates relationships before it produces conclusions. It identifies variables, tests how they interact, and builds an output that follows from those interactions. The process is constrained by the structure of the problem. Each step must maintain continuity with the input and remain consistent with observed outcomes. This constraint limits which conclusions can persist because any mismatch between the model and reality is exposed through feedback.

Narrative-driven reasoning operates under a different constraint. Instead of constructing conclusions from relationships, the system organizes inputs into a sequence that forms a coherent story. Events are arranged in a way that produces continuity, causation is inferred from temporal order, and gaps are filled with assumptions that preserve flow. The output is not evaluated based on whether it accurately represents underlying relationships. It is evaluated based on whether the sequence feels complete and internally consistent. A conclusion is accepted when it resolves the narrative, not when it has been derived from tested interactions between variables.

This shift changes how causality is assigned. In a structured system, causality is determined by examining whether a change in one variable produces a consistent change in another under controlled conditions. The relationship must hold across multiple instances to be considered valid. In a narrative system, causality is often inferred from proximity. If one event follows another and the sequence can be arranged into a coherent progression, the system treats the earlier event as the cause of the later one. This reduces the need for validation. The story provides an explanation that appears sufficient because it maintains continuity.

Narrative reasoning compresses complexity by reducing multiple interacting variables into a single linear pathway. Real systems often involve overlapping processes that operate simultaneously and influence each other in non-linear ways. A narrative selects a subset of these variables and arranges them into a sequence that can be followed from beginning to end. This makes the problem easier to process, but it removes interactions that may be critical to understanding the outcome. The resulting explanation is simpler, but it is not structurally complete.

As narrative becomes the dominant mode, the system begins to prioritize coherence over accuracy. Information that fits into the existing story is integrated because it strengthens continuity. Information that disrupts the sequence is modified or excluded because it introduces breaks that would require restructuring the narrative. This filtering process allows the system to maintain a stable story even when the underlying conditions do not support it. The model becomes organized around maintaining the narrative rather than aligning with external structure.

This mode of reasoning also reduces traceability. A narrative provides a sequence of events, but it does not expose the underlying relationships that produced those events. When an outcome is incorrect, the system can adjust the story by altering elements within the sequence, but it cannot identify which specific relationship failed because those relationships were never explicitly represented. Correction occurs at the level of the narrative rather than at the level of the mechanism.

Over time, the system develops a preference for explanations that are easy to follow. Simplicity in presentation becomes a proxy for correctness. Explanations that require multiple interacting variables or non-linear relationships are avoided because they do not translate into a clean sequence. The system selects interpretations that can be expressed as a clear progression from cause to effect, even when the actual structure of the problem does not support that progression. This introduces systematic distortion. The model reflects the constraints of the narrative rather than the structure of the environment.

Narrative reasoning does not eliminate logical capacity. It overlays it with a framework that organizes outputs into sequences that are easier to process. The system can still engage in structured analysis, but it is less likely to do so when a narrative provides a sufficient explanation to satisfy internal constraints. This reduces the frequency of deeper evaluation and allows untested assumptions to persist within the model.

Restoring logical structure requires separating explanation from validation. The system must evaluate relationships independently of how they are presented. Variables must be defined, interactions must be tested, and conclusions must be derived from those interactions before they are arranged into any form of narrative. When this sequence is maintained, stories can be used to communicate results, but they do not determine them. The model remains anchored to the structure of the problem, and the narrative becomes a representation of that structure rather than a substitute for it.

Authority and Familiarity Bias

A structured thinking system verifies claims by testing their relationship to observable outcomes. Inputs are not accepted based on origin. They are evaluated by how well they map to conditions that can be measured, predicted, and reproduced. This requires the system to construct a model, generate expectations, and compare those expectations against results. Verification is therefore an internal process. External information can initiate it, but it does not complete it. Accuracy depends on whether the system can confirm that a claim corresponds to reality through its own evaluation.

Authority and familiarity introduce an alternative pathway. Instead of verifying a claim through direct evaluation, the system uses the source of the claim or its prior exposure as a proxy for correctness. Information from a recognized authority is accepted because it has been associated with reliability in the past. Information that feels familiar is accepted because it has been encountered repeatedly and integrated into existing patterns. In both cases, the system bypasses the verification step. It replaces the relationship between claim and outcome with a relationship between claim and source.

This substitution reduces computational cost. Verification requires building and testing a model, which consumes time and resources. Relying on authority or familiarity allows the system to accept information immediately without reconstructing the underlying relationships. Under conditions of high input volume or time pressure, this pathway becomes efficient. It allows the system to process large amounts of information without exceeding its capacity. However, the efficiency comes from removing the constraint that ensures accuracy. The claim is accepted without being tied to external conditions that would confirm or contradict it.

Authority functions as a compression mechanism. A source that has produced accurate information in the past becomes a container for future claims. The system assigns a higher probability of correctness to new information from that source, reducing the need for independent evaluation. This can be effective when the authority's outputs remain aligned with reality, but it introduces systemic risk. If the source produces an incorrect claim, the system is less likely to detect it because it has reduced its verification effort. The error passes through the system with the same weight as a validated conclusion.

Familiarity operates through repetition. Each exposure to a claim strengthens its presence within the system. The claim becomes easier to retrieve and integrates more tightly with existing patterns. Over time, this ease of access is interpreted as evidence of correctness. The system treats the claim as stable because it is consistently available, not because it has been tested. This creates a feedback loop. Repeated exposure increases acceptance, and acceptance increases the likelihood of further exposure, reinforcing the pattern without reference to external validation.

Both mechanisms shift the reference point of the system outward. Instead of evaluating whether a claim aligns with observable outcomes, the system evaluates whether it aligns with recognized sources or established patterns. This changes how contradictions are handled. When new information conflicts with an authority, the system is more likely to reject the new information or reinterpret it to preserve the authority's position. When new information conflicts with familiar patterns, it is treated as an exception or anomaly rather than a signal that the model requires adjustment.

This shift reduces traceability. In a verification-driven system, each conclusion can be linked to a set of relationships that have been tested against outcomes. When authority or familiarity replaces verification, the pathway from input to conclusion is shortened. The system can state that a claim is accepted, but it cannot reconstruct the reasoning that connects it to reality because that reasoning was never performed. When an error is discovered, the system lacks a defined location within the process where correction can occur. It may reduce reliance on a specific source or adjust its exposure patterns, but it cannot directly modify the relationship between the claim and the underlying conditions.

Over time, the accumulation of unverified inputs alters the structure of the model. The system integrates claims that have not been tested, and these claims interact with each other to produce further conclusions. Because the underlying relationships have not been validated, the model becomes sensitive to inconsistencies that are not immediately visible. It may function under familiar conditions where the unverified claims happen to align with reality, but it becomes unstable when conditions change or when conflicting information is introduced.

The reliance on external anchors does not remove the system's capacity to verify. It reduces the frequency with which verification is used. The system defaults to accepting information based on source or familiarity because it is more efficient, especially in environments that reward rapid processing. Verification becomes selective rather than continuous. It is applied only when contradictions become too large to ignore, at which point the cost of correction is higher because multiple unverified elements are embedded within the model.

Restoring verification requires reestablishing the link between claims and outcomes. Information must be evaluated based on its correspondence to observable conditions rather than its source or repetition. This does not eliminate the use of authority or familiarity as preliminary filters, but it prevents them from determining acceptance. The system must reconstruct the pathway from input to conclusion, test the relationships involved, and confirm that the output holds under varying conditions. When verification is active, external anchors lose their ability to override accuracy, and the model remains aligned with the structure it is intended to represent.

Chapter 4

Accumulation Failure

A thinking system builds its capacity over time by retaining validated structure. Each correct relationship that is established and reinforced becomes part of the model that future decisions depend on. This accumulation is not simply storage. It is integration. New inputs are not kept as isolated pieces of information. They are connected to existing relationships, allowing the system to expand its representation of reality while maintaining coherence. When this process functions correctly, the system becomes more accurate as it gains experience because each addition strengthens the underlying architecture.

Accumulation failure occurs when new inputs are added without being properly integrated into the structure of the model. The system continues to gather information, but it does not convert that information into usable relationships. Inputs remain fragmented. They exist as separate elements that can be recalled, but they do not interact with each other in a way that improves predictive accuracy. The system appears to be increasing in knowledge because the volume of stored information grows, but the functional capacity of the model does not improve at the same rate.

This breakdown begins when validation is reduced or removed. For information to be integrated, the system must determine how it relates to existing components. This requires testing whether the new input aligns with or contradicts the current model and adjusting the structure accordingly. When inputs are accepted without this process, they are stored without defined relationships. The system accumulates data points, but it does not establish the connections that would allow those data points to inform future decisions.

Fragmentation introduces instability. When the system attempts to use its stored information, it must select which elements are relevant to the current problem. In a well-integrated model, relevance is determined by structured relationships. The system can identify which variables interact and how they influence the outcome. In a fragmented model, relevance is determined by accessibility or similarity. The system retrieves information that appears related based on surface features rather than structural connection. This increases the probability that the retrieved information does not correspond to the actual requirements of the problem.

As accumulation continues without integration, the model becomes saturated with unstructured inputs. Each new piece of information increases the number of possible combinations that the system can form, but without defined relationships, these combinations are not constrained. The system must navigate a larger space of possibilities with fewer structural guides. This reduces efficiency and accuracy. Decisions require more effort to produce because the system must sort through a greater volume of unconnected elements, yet the outputs remain imprecise because the relationships between those elements are not defined.

Accumulation failure also affects how contradictions are handled. In an integrated system, conflicting information triggers a restructuring process. The system identifies the inconsistency, evaluates which components are inaccurate, and adjusts the model to resolve the conflict. In a fragmented system, contradictions can coexist because the elements involved are not tightly connected. The system can hold multiple incompatible inputs without detecting the inconsistency, because there is no structure forcing those inputs to interact. This allows errors to persist without being exposed.

Over time, the presence of unintegrated information degrades the reliability of the model. The system may retrieve correct elements, but it combines them with unrelated or incorrect elements because it lacks a framework for determining how they should interact. Outputs become inconsistent. The same problem may produce different results depending on which fragments are activated. The system's performance becomes unpredictable because it is not operating on a stable set of relationships.

The accumulation of unstructured inputs also increases cognitive load. The system must manage a growing volume of information without the benefit of compression that comes from integration. In a structured model, multiple inputs can be represented through a smaller set of relationships that capture their interactions. In a fragmented model, each input must be considered individually. This increases the effort required to process information and reduces the system's ability to handle complex problems efficiently.

This failure mode is reinforced by environments that reward information acquisition without requiring integration. The system receives continuous input and is encouraged to store it, but it is not required to test or connect that input to existing structure. Over time, the act of accumulation becomes decoupled from the act of building a model. The system measures progress by the amount of information it holds rather than by the accuracy of its predictions.

Restoring accumulation requires converting stored inputs into structured relationships. Each new piece of information must be evaluated in the context of the existing model, determining how it interacts with known variables and whether it modifies those relationships. Contradictions must be resolved through restructuring rather than tolerated as separate fragments. As integration increases, the system compresses information into a form that is easier to process and more useful for prediction. Accumulation becomes functional again because it strengthens the architecture rather than expanding unstructured storage.

Decisions as Trajectories

A decision is not an isolated event. It is an initiation point that sets a direction within a system that continues to evolve after the choice is made. Once an action is taken, it alters the state of the system. Resources are allocated, constraints are introduced, and future options are reshaped by the new configuration. Each subsequent decision is made from within this altered state rather than from the original baseline. This creates continuity. Decisions link together, forming a trajectory that reflects the structure of the model that produced them.

When the underlying model is accurate, this continuity produces alignment. Each decision reinforces a direction that corresponds to external conditions. The system adjusts as it moves, but the adjustments occur within a trajectory that remains close to the structure it is interacting with. Small errors are corrected through feedback, preventing deviation from accumulating. The path may shift, but it does not diverge. The system maintains coherence between its internal representation and the environment because each step is evaluated and adjusted as it occurs.

When the model is misaligned, the same continuity produces a different outcome. The initial decision sets a direction that does not correspond to the underlying structure of the environment. Because future decisions are made from within the state created by prior ones, the system continues to operate along this incorrect path. Each new decision compounds the deviation. The system is not only moving away from alignment. It is doing so within a framework that reinforces the direction of that movement.

The compounding effect is driven by dependency. Early decisions determine the range of available options for later decisions. When those early decisions are based on inaccurate assumptions, they constrain the system in ways that reflect those inaccuracies. As the system progresses, it becomes increasingly committed to the trajectory it has established. Reversing direction requires overcoming the constraints created by prior actions, which often involves higher cost than continuing forward. This creates inertia. The system continues along the existing path even when evidence begins to indicate that the path is incorrect.

Time amplifies this process. The longer the system operates on a misaligned trajectory, the more layers of decisions accumulate on top of the original error. Each layer adds complexity, making it more difficult to isolate the point where the misalignment began. The system experiences the effects as present-state problems without clear visibility into their origin. Correction becomes less precise because the deviation is distributed across multiple decisions rather than localized to a single point.

Feedback can interrupt this trajectory, but only if it is strong enough and received early enough to trigger adjustment. When feedback is delayed or ambiguous, the system does not detect the misalignment at the stage where correction would be most efficient. It continues to build on the existing trajectory, increasing the cost of change. By the time the discrepancy becomes clear, the system has committed significant resources to the path, and reversing it requires restructuring multiple layers of prior decisions.

As misalignment compounds, the system may attempt to stabilize by adjusting surface-level behavior. It modifies individual decisions in response to immediate outcomes without addressing the underlying model that is generating those decisions. This can produce temporary improvements, but it does not correct the trajectory. The system remains oriented in the wrong direction, and the adjustments only slow the rate of divergence rather than eliminating it.

Trajectory-based thinking reveals that accuracy at the point of decision has effects that extend beyond the immediate outcome. A single incorrect assumption can influence a sequence of decisions that follow, each one reinforcing the initial error. Conversely, a correct assumption can guide multiple decisions in a direction that maintains alignment with external conditions. The impact of a decision is therefore not limited to its direct result. It includes the structure it imposes on future choices.

Maintaining alignment requires continuous correction at each step in the trajectory. The system must evaluate not only whether a decision produced the expected outcome, but whether the direction it is moving remains consistent with external conditions. This requires feedback that is both timely and specific enough to identify deviations early. When small errors are corrected immediately, they do not accumulate. The trajectory remains stable because it is continuously adjusted to reflect the structure it is navigating.

When correction is absent or ineffective, misalignment becomes embedded in the trajectory itself. The system continues to function, but its path diverges further with each step. The divergence is not random. It is the result of consistent decisions made within a misaligned model. Over time, the gap between the system's direction and the structure of the environment becomes large enough that outcomes degrade in a way that can no longer be compensated for through local adjustments.

Reestablishing alignment requires identifying the trajectory rather than focusing solely on individual decisions. The system must examine how prior choices have shaped its current state and determine whether the direction implied by those choices corresponds to external conditions. Correction may require reversing or restructuring earlier decisions to change the path of the system. This is more costly than adjusting a single action, but it is necessary when misalignment has compounded across multiple steps. When the trajectory is corrected, subsequent decisions begin to reinforce alignment again, and the system regains stability as it moves forward.

Invisible Costs of Poor Thinking

Poor thinking rarely produces immediate failure. A flawed decision can generate an outcome that appears acceptable within the current time window, especially when feedback is delayed or filtered through multiple variables. The system registers the result as neutral or even positive, and the underlying model remains unchanged. This creates the initial condition for divergence. The decision did not align with the structure of the environment, but the misalignment was not exposed at the point where correction could occur.

The cost emerges over time as the effects of that decision propagate through subsequent states of the system. Each decision alters the configuration of resources, constraints, and available options. When the initial decision is based on an inaccurate model, it introduces a distortion into that configuration. Future decisions are then made within this distorted state, carrying the error forward. The system continues to operate, but the path it follows begins to deviate from one that would maintain alignment with external conditions.

Delayed divergence is driven by accumulation. A single misaligned decision may not produce a noticeable difference, but repeated decisions based on the same flawed structure compound the deviation. Each step adds a small increment of error, and those increments interact. The system does not experience this as a single event. It experiences it as a gradual shift in outcomes that becomes more pronounced over time. Early signals are weak and often indistinguishable from normal variability, so they do not trigger correction.

The invisibility of the cost is maintained by short-term stability. Many environments allow inaccurate models to function for extended periods because they do not immediately penalize misalignment. Buffers absorb the impact. Redundant pathways compensate for inefficiencies. External support structures maintain output even when internal processes are suboptimal. These factors allow the system to continue producing acceptable results while the underlying model drifts. The absence of immediate negative feedback reinforces the use of the flawed structure.

As divergence progresses, the system begins to encounter outcomes that do not match its expectations. At first, these are treated as isolated anomalies. The system adjusts locally, modifying individual decisions to address specific issues without examining the underlying model. This maintains short-term performance but does not correct the trajectory. The source of the divergence remains embedded in the structure, continuing to influence future decisions.

Over time, the discrepancy between expected and actual outcomes becomes consistent. The system's predictions lose reliability. Variability increases because the model no longer captures the relationships that determine results. At this stage, the cost becomes visible, but it is difficult to attribute. The effects are distributed across multiple decisions and time periods. There is no single point where the failure can be isolated because the divergence developed incrementally.

Delayed divergence also increases the cost of correction. Early in the process, a small adjustment to the model would realign the system with minimal disruption. As divergence accumulates, more components of the system become dependent on the misaligned structure. Correcting the model requires restructuring these components, which involves higher resource expenditure and greater disruption to ongoing processes. The system faces a tradeoff between continuing on a flawed path with increasing cost or incurring the immediate cost of restructuring to restore alignment.

The perception of stability during the early stages of divergence creates a bias toward continuation. Because the system appears to function, there is no immediate incentive to question the underlying model. The cost remains hidden until it reaches a threshold where it can no longer be absorbed. At that point, the system experiences a sharper decline in performance, not because the error is new, but because the accumulated effects have exceeded the capacity of buffers and compensatory mechanisms.

Delayed divergence demonstrates that the quality of thinking cannot be evaluated solely by immediate outcomes. A decision must be assessed based on whether it aligns with the structure that governs long-term results. This requires examining the relationships that produced the decision rather than relying on the short-term outcome as evidence of correctness. Without this evaluation, the system is vulnerable to accumulating errors that remain undetected until they produce significant impact.

Preventing invisible costs requires early detection of misalignment. The system must maintain feedback mechanisms that can identify small discrepancies between prediction and outcome before they accumulate. It must evaluate the trajectory of its decisions rather than individual results, ensuring that each step maintains alignment with external conditions. When correction occurs at this stage, divergence is limited, and the cost remains low. When correction is delayed, the system continues to operate under a flawed model until the accumulated deviation forces a more costly adjustment.

System Drift and Outcome Collapse

A system does not fail at the moment outcomes collapse. It fails when its internal structure loses alignment with the conditions that determine those outcomes. The visible breakdown is a late-stage expression of a process that has been unfolding over time. Drift begins at the level of relationships within the model. Variables are misrepresented, interactions are simplified or omitted, and feedback is either delayed or misinterpreted. Each of these changes is small enough to avoid immediate disruption. The system continues to function because the remaining structure is sufficient to produce acceptable outputs under current conditions.

Drift accumulates through repeated operation under a misaligned model. Each cycle of decision and outcome reinforces the existing structure, even when that structure does not correspond to reality. The system adapts to its own outputs. It adjusts behavior locally to maintain performance, but these adjustments occur within the constraints of the misaligned model. They do not correct the underlying relationships. Instead, they create compensatory layers that allow the system to continue operating despite increasing deviation.

As these layers accumulate, the system becomes more complex but less stable. The internal model no longer reflects a single coherent structure. It becomes a collection of adjustments that interact in ways that are not fully understood or explicitly represented. This reduces predictability. The system can still produce correct outputs in familiar conditions where compensations are sufficient, but it becomes sensitive to changes that were previously manageable. Small variations in input begin to produce larger variations in output because the structure that once stabilized those relationships has degraded.

The appearance of stability during drift is maintained by buffering. External systems absorb variability, internal redundancies compensate for inefficiencies, and delayed feedback prevents immediate exposure of errors. These mechanisms extend the functional life of the system, but they also allow misalignment to deepen. Because failure is not immediate, there is no clear signal indicating that the structure requires correction. The system continues to operate, and the absence of visible breakdown reinforces the assumption that the model remains valid.

Outcome collapse occurs when the system reaches a point where compensatory mechanisms can no longer maintain function. This threshold is not defined by a single event. It is defined by the cumulative effect of drift across multiple components. As misalignment increases, the system's ability to absorb variability decreases. Inputs that were previously within tolerance begin to exceed the system's capacity to respond. The internal adjustments that once stabilized performance become insufficient, and the system can no longer produce outputs that align with expectations.

The transition from apparent stability to visible failure appears sudden because the system has been operating near this threshold for some time. The final change that precedes collapse may be small, but it occurs in a context where the margin for error has been reduced. The system no longer has the structural integrity required to absorb even minor deviations. When this limit is reached, outcomes shift rapidly because the underlying support that maintained stability is no longer present.

This pattern obscures the origin of failure. The system experiences the collapse as a recent event, but the structural causes are distributed across prior decisions and adjustments. There is no single point where the failure began. It is embedded in the gradual drift that occurred over time. This makes post-collapse analysis difficult. The system may identify the immediate trigger, but that trigger only reveals the final stage of a longer process.

Drift also reduces the system's ability to correct itself before collapse. As the model becomes more misaligned, feedback signals become less reliable. The system cannot accurately interpret outcomes because its representation of the relationships that produced those outcomes is already degraded. Attempts to adjust may target symptoms rather than causes, further complicating the structure without restoring alignment. This accelerates the approach to collapse because the system adds layers of adjustment that do not resolve the underlying issue.

The sudden appearance of failure is therefore a property of accumulated structural degradation. The system remains functional while drift is within the range that compensatory mechanisms can absorb. Once that range is exceeded, the system transitions rapidly to a state where outputs no longer match expectations. The change is abrupt in appearance but continuous in origin.

Preventing outcome collapse requires maintaining alignment at the structural level before drift accumulates. The system must preserve clear relationships between variables, ensure that feedback remains accurate and timely, and limit the use of compensatory adjustments that mask underlying misalignment. When discrepancies are detected, they must be resolved by updating the model rather than by layering additional mechanisms to maintain short-term performance. This keeps the system within a range where stability is supported by accurate structure rather than by temporary compensation, reducing the likelihood that drift will reach a point where collapse becomes inevitable.

PART II

THE STRUCTURE OF LOGIC

Chapter 5

What Logic Is

Logic is not a set of rules applied after thinking. It is the structure that determines whether thinking can produce outputs that correspond to reality. A system does not become logical by following formal steps in isolation. It becomes logical when the relationships between its internal representations match the relationships present in the environment it is operating within. Logic is therefore not an abstract layer added to cognition. It is the architecture that binds inputs, transformations, and outputs into a continuous structure where each element constrains the next.

At its core, logic is the preservation of relationships across transformation. An input enters the system in some form, is converted into an internal representation, and then manipulated to produce an output. For that output to remain aligned with reality, the relationships that existed in the input must be preserved through each stage of this process. If a relationship is altered, omitted, or replaced without justification, the output no longer reflects the structure it was derived from. The system may still produce a coherent answer, but that answer will not correspond to the conditions it is meant to represent.

This preservation requires explicit representation of variables and their interactions. A system cannot maintain relationships it does not define. Variables must be identified, their boundaries must be clear, and the ways in which they influence each other must be specified. Logic emerges when these definitions are stable and when transformations operate on them without introducing distortion. Each step in the reasoning process must maintain continuity with the previous step, ensuring that the structure is carried forward rather than reconstructed from approximation.

Relational structure imposes constraint. It limits the set of possible conclusions to those that can be derived from the defined relationships. This is not a restriction that reduces capability. It is the mechanism that prevents error from propagating. Without constraint, the system can move from input to output through arbitrary pathways that are not tied to the structure of the problem. With constraint, each transition must be justified by the relationships that have been established. This ensures that the output remains anchored to the input rather than drifting into internally coherent but externally inaccurate conclusions.

The stability of logic depends on traceability. Each output must be linked to the sequence of transformations that produced it. This linkage allows the system to inspect its own process and identify where relationships may have been altered incorrectly. When an error is detected, the system can return to the specific point in the sequence where the mismatch occurred and adjust the relationship at that location. Without traceability, correction becomes imprecise because the system cannot determine which part of the structure failed.

Logic also depends on consistency across contexts. A relationship that holds under one set of conditions must hold under similar conditions unless a defined variable changes. This allows the system to generalize its model without losing accuracy. When relationships are stable, the system can apply them to new inputs with confidence that the resulting outputs will remain aligned. When relationships are inconsistent or undefined, the system cannot predict how changes in input will affect the output, and reasoning becomes unreliable.

This framework distinguishes logic from heuristic or narrative processes. Heuristics compress relationships into patterns, allowing rapid response but reducing explicit representation. Narratives organize outputs into sequences that maintain coherence but do not necessarily preserve underlying interactions. Both can produce usable outputs, but neither guarantees that the relationships between variables have been maintained. Logic requires that those relationships be defined, preserved, and traceable at every stage.

The system that operates on relational structure does not rely on correctness emerging by chance. It enforces conditions under which correct outputs are the natural result of the process. When the architecture is intact, accuracy becomes repeatable because each step in the process maintains alignment with the structure it represents. When the architecture is degraded, outputs may still appear correct, but they do so without a mechanism that ensures consistency across different inputs and conditions.

Understanding logic as relational structure shifts the focus from producing answers to maintaining architecture. The system must prioritize the integrity of the relationships it uses to process information. Inputs must be decomposed into variables, interactions must be explicitly defined, and transformations must preserve those interactions without distortion. When this is done, the output is not an isolated result. It is the final state of a sequence that has maintained alignment from beginning to end, and that sequence can be examined, adjusted, and reused across contexts without losing its connection to reality.

Structure vs Content

A thinking system operates on two distinct layers. Content provides the raw material, while structure determines how that material is processed. Inputs enter as data, observations, or claims. Structure defines how those inputs are represented, how relationships between them are established, and how conclusions are produced. The output of the system is not determined by content alone. It is the result of how content is transformed within the structure. When structure is accurate, even incomplete inputs can be organized into a model that improves over time through correction. When structure is degraded, even high-quality inputs are processed in ways that produce distortion.

Correct reasoning depends on the preservation of relationships during transformation. Inputs must be decomposed into variables, those variables must be connected through defined interactions, and each step in the process must maintain continuity with the previous one. This ensures that the output reflects the structure present in the input rather than an approximation derived from pattern or familiarity. If structure is intact, the system can detect gaps in content because missing variables disrupt the relationships required to complete the model. This creates a signal that drives further inquiry or prevents premature conclusions.

Content without structure does not produce reliable outcomes. A system can possess accurate information and still generate incorrect conclusions if it lacks the architecture to process that information properly. Inputs may be recalled correctly, but if their relationships are not defined or preserved, they are combined in ways that do not correspond to reality. The system appears informed because it can access correct data, but its outputs are inconsistent because that data is not integrated into a coherent model. The error does not originate in the input. It originates in the transformation.

Structure without content produces a different limitation. The system maintains defined relationships and can process inputs in a way that preserves those relationships, but the model remains incomplete if critical variables are absent. In this case, reasoning remains stable, but its scope is limited. The system can generate accurate conclusions within the range of the inputs it possesses, but it cannot account for factors that have not been represented. The absence of content introduces uncertainty, but it does not distort the relationships that are present. This allows the system to recognize the limits of its model rather than producing confident but inaccurate outputs.

The interaction between structure and content determines how error is introduced and how it propagates. When content is incorrect but structure is intact, the system can detect inconsistency through feedback. Outcomes will not match predictions, and the system can trace the mismatch back to the specific input that is inaccurate. Correction is localized. The incorrect element is replaced or adjusted, and the rest of the structure remains stable. When structure is degraded, this localization is lost. Errors in content interact with errors in transformation, producing outputs that cannot be traced back to a single source. Correction becomes diffuse because the system cannot distinguish between flaws in input and flaws in processing.

Over time, systems that prioritize content over structure accumulate information without improving accuracy. They expand the volume of inputs they can access, but they do not increase their ability to organize those inputs into reliable models. This creates an illusion of progress. The system appears more knowledgeable, but its predictions do not become more consistent because the underlying architecture has not improved. In contrast, systems that prioritize structure can operate effectively even with limited content. They maintain alignment because each input is processed in a way that preserves relationships, allowing the model to refine itself as new information is added.

The distinction also determines how the system responds to new inputs. In a structure-driven system, new information is evaluated based on how it interacts with existing relationships. It is integrated if it aligns or triggers restructuring if it introduces contradiction. In a content-driven system, new information is added without this evaluation. It increases the volume of stored data, but it does not necessarily improve the model. Contradictions can accumulate because there is no mechanism forcing inputs to interact within a consistent framework.

Maintaining correct reasoning requires prioritizing structure as the primary constraint. Content must be processed through defined relationships that are preserved across each step of transformation. This allows the system to remain aligned even as inputs change. When structure is stable, content becomes functional because it can be integrated into a model that produces consistent outputs. When structure is unstable, content remains fragmented, and the system cannot reliably convert information into accurate conclusions.

The system that recognizes this distinction does not attempt to solve problems by acquiring more data alone. It ensures that the architecture used to process that data can maintain relationships without distortion. Inputs are then added into a framework that can evaluate, integrate, and correct them. This produces a model that improves over time because both structure and content are aligned. The output reflects not just what the system knows, but how well it can preserve the relationships that define what is true.

Alignment With Reality

A thinking system can produce outputs that are internally valid without those outputs corresponding to external conditions. Internal validity refers to consistency within the model. The relationships between variables do not contradict each other, and conclusions follow from the assumptions that have been defined. This creates a closed structure that can generate stable outputs. However, stability within the system does not guarantee that those outputs map to reality. The model may be coherent, but if its assumptions or relationships do not reflect actual conditions, the conclusions it produces will diverge from what occurs outside the system.

External truth is determined by correspondence. A model aligns with reality when its structure produces predictions that match observed outcomes across varying conditions. This requires that the relationships defined within the system mirror the relationships that govern the environment. Internal consistency is necessary for this alignment, but it is not sufficient. A model can be internally consistent while still being constructed on incorrect premises or incomplete representations. In such cases, the system will generate conclusions that appear correct within its own framework but fail when tested against real-world conditions.

The distinction becomes clear at the point of validation. Internal validity is assessed by examining whether the system's conclusions follow logically from its premises. External truth is assessed by comparing those conclusions to outcomes that exist independently of the system. When a model is aligned, these two evaluations converge. Conclusions that are internally consistent also produce accurate predictions. When the model is misaligned, the evaluations diverge. The system can produce internally valid conclusions that do not correspond to observed results.

Misalignment often persists because internal validity is easier to maintain. The system has direct access to its own structure and can resolve inconsistencies by adjusting assumptions or redefining relationships. This process does not require external reference. It allows the system to stabilize itself without confronting discrepancies between its model and reality. External validation requires comparison with outcomes that are not controlled by the system. It introduces constraints that cannot be modified to preserve internal coherence. When feedback is weak or delayed, the system may default to maintaining internal validity because it is more immediately accessible.

This shift alters how errors are handled. In a system focused on internal validity, error appears as contradiction within the model. Correction involves restoring consistency by modifying elements until the contradiction is resolved. In a system focused on external truth, error appears as a mismatch between prediction and outcome. Correction involves identifying which part of the model failed to correspond to reality and adjusting that component. These processes are not interchangeable. A system can eliminate internal contradictions without improving its alignment with external conditions if it does not test its assumptions against outcomes.

The relationship between internal validity and external truth determines how the system evolves over time. When external alignment is maintained, the model is continuously updated through feedback. Assumptions that do not produce accurate predictions are replaced, and relationships are refined. The system converges toward a structure that reflects the environment. When internal validity is prioritized without external testing, the model evolves based on its own constraints. It becomes more coherent internally but may drift further from reality because its updates are not anchored to outcomes.

Alignment requires maintaining both properties in sequence rather than in isolation. Internal validity ensures that the model operates without contradiction. External validation ensures that the model corresponds to conditions outside itself. The system must first construct relationships that are consistent and then test those relationships against outcomes. If a mismatch occurs, the model must be revised even if it disrupts internal coherence. This process may introduce temporary instability within the system, but it is necessary to restore alignment with external structure.

The failure to maintain this sequence leads to a system that can justify its conclusions without verifying them. It produces outputs that are logically consistent within its own framework but do not reliably predict or explain real-world behavior. This creates a separation between what the system believes and what actually occurs. Over time, the gap widens as the model continues to evolve based on internal constraints rather than external correction.

Restoring alignment requires reestablishing outcome-based validation as the final constraint. The system must treat correspondence with reality as the determining factor in whether a model is correct. Internal validity remains necessary, but it must serve as a foundation for testing rather than a substitute for it. When both properties are maintained, the system produces outputs that are not only consistent within the model but also accurate in relation to the environment. This convergence is what allows reasoning to function as a reliable mechanism for navigating and predicting real conditions.

Chapter 6

Language and Precision

A thinking system operates through representations, and language is the primary medium through which those representations are formed, stored, and manipulated. Words are not neutral labels attached to ideas. They define the boundaries of variables, determine how relationships are expressed, and constrain what distinctions the system is capable of making. When language is precise, the system can isolate components, track interactions, and maintain continuity across transformations. When language is imprecise, variables blur, relationships collapse into approximations, and the structure required for accurate reasoning degrades at the point of representation.

Precision begins with definition. A variable must have clear boundaries so that it can be distinguished from other variables and tracked consistently across contexts. If a term shifts meaning depending on how it is used, the system cannot maintain stable relationships because it is not operating on a fixed object. The same word may refer to different underlying structures, or different words may refer to the same structure without explicit recognition. This introduces ambiguity into every stage of reasoning. The system processes inputs that appear consistent at the surface level, but the underlying variables are not aligned, leading to outputs that do not preserve the intended relationships.

Language also determines how relationships are encoded. The connections between variables must be expressed in a way that reflects their actual interaction. If language compresses or generalizes these relationships, it removes detail that may be critical for maintaining accuracy. For example, describing a process as "affecting" another variable does not specify the direction, magnitude, or conditions under which the interaction occurs. This leaves the relationship underdefined. The system may treat it as stable across contexts when it is not, or fail to recognize conditions where the relationship changes. Precision requires that relationships be described in a way that preserves their structure rather than approximating it.

As reasoning progresses, language must maintain continuity. Each transformation from input to output depends on the consistent use of terms and relationships. If a variable is redefined mid-process or if a relationship is altered without explicit acknowledgment, the system loses track of what is being manipulated. The output may still appear coherent, but it is no longer derived from the same structure that defined the input. This breaks traceability. The system cannot reconstruct how the conclusion was formed because the representations changed during the process.

Imprecision in language also affects error detection. When variables are clearly defined and relationships are explicit, mismatches between prediction and outcome can be traced to specific components of the model. The system can identify which variable was misrepresented or which interaction was incorrect and adjust accordingly. When language is ambiguous, errors cannot be localized. The system cannot determine whether the issue lies in the definition of a variable, the expression of a relationship, or the transformation applied during reasoning. Correction becomes broad and inefficient because the source of the error is not identifiable.

Compression is a common source of imprecision. To reduce cognitive load, the system often condenses complex structures into single terms or simplified descriptions. While this increases efficiency, it removes internal detail. A compressed term may represent multiple variables and interactions without exposing them. When the system uses this term in reasoning, it operates on an abstraction rather than on the underlying structure. This can produce acceptable results in familiar contexts where the abstraction aligns with reality, but it reduces adaptability. When conditions change, the system lacks the detail required to adjust its model accurately.

The relationship between language and precision also determines how new information is integrated. Precise language allows new inputs to be mapped onto existing variables and relationships with minimal distortion. The system can identify where the new information fits and how it modifies the model. Imprecise language forces the system to approximate this mapping. New inputs may be assigned to existing terms that do not fully capture their structure, or they may create redundant representations that fragment the model. This reduces the system's ability to maintain a coherent and integrated structure over time.

Precision does not require complexity in presentation. It requires accuracy in representation. A system can use simple language if that language maintains clear definitions and preserves relationships. Complexity arises when multiple variables and interactions must be represented simultaneously, but the principle remains the same. Each element must be defined, and each relationship must be expressed in a way that can be consistently applied. The goal is not to increase the number of terms, but to ensure that each term corresponds to a distinct and stable component of the model.

As precision increases, the system gains control over its own reasoning. It can manipulate variables without losing track of their identity, adjust relationships without introducing unintended distortion, and trace outputs back to their origin within the model. This control allows for targeted correction and consistent application across contexts. Without precision, the system operates on shifting representations, and its outputs become dependent on approximation rather than structure.

Maintaining precision requires continuous attention to how language is used within the system. Definitions must be established and preserved. Relationships must be expressed with sufficient detail to reflect actual interactions. Transformations must operate on stable representations without redefining them implicitly. When these conditions are met, language becomes a tool that supports accurate reasoning. When they are not, language becomes a source of distortion that undermines the system's ability to maintain alignment with the structure it is attempting to represent.

Definitions as Boundaries

A thinking system operates on discrete units that must remain stable as they are moved through different stages of reasoning. Definitions establish the boundaries of those units. They determine what is included within a variable and what is excluded, allowing the system to treat that variable as a consistent object across contexts. Without defined boundaries, the system cannot preserve identity. A term may appear the same at the surface level, but if its underlying meaning shifts during processing, the system is no longer operating on a fixed element. This introduces distortion at the point of representation, and that distortion propagates through every subsequent transformation.

Concept stability depends on boundary integrity. A variable must maintain its definition as it interacts with other variables. If its scope expands or contracts without explicit recognition, the relationships built upon it lose coherence. For example, a term that initially refers to a specific process may later be used to describe a broader category that includes additional components. The system treats these uses as equivalent because the label has not changed, but the underlying structure has. This creates hidden inconsistency. The system appears to be reasoning within a single framework, but it is actually shifting between different definitions of the same term.

Boundaries also determine how variables interact. Relationships between variables are only valid if the variables themselves are clearly defined. If a boundary is ambiguous, the system cannot specify how one variable influences another because it does not know what is being affected. This leads to generalized relationships that lack precision. The system may describe interactions in broad terms, but those descriptions do not preserve the structure required for accurate prediction. The output reflects an approximation of the relationship rather than a defined interaction.

As reasoning progresses, stable definitions allow the system to maintain continuity. Each step in the process builds on the previous one, and that continuity depends on the consistent use of variables. If a variable is redefined mid-process, the system loses track of what has been established. The conclusion may still follow from the steps taken, but those steps are no longer connected to the original input in a consistent way. Traceability is lost because the pathway from input to output involves shifting representations rather than stable elements.

Imprecise boundaries also interfere with error detection. When a prediction does not match an outcome, the system must identify which part of the model failed. If variables are clearly defined, the system can isolate the discrepancy to a specific component. If boundaries are unstable, the system cannot determine whether the error originates from the variable itself or from the relationship applied to it. Correction becomes diffuse. The system may adjust multiple elements without resolving the underlying issue because it cannot localize the source of the mismatch.

Compression increases the risk of boundary instability. Complex structures are often reduced to single terms to simplify processing. This reduction removes internal detail and expands the scope of the term to cover multiple components. The system gains efficiency, but it loses precision. When the compressed term is used in reasoning, the system cannot distinguish between the components it represents. This prevents accurate mapping of relationships because the variable no longer corresponds to a single defined structure. It corresponds to a collection of elements that may behave differently under different conditions.

Stable definitions allow for integration. New information can be incorporated into the model by mapping it onto existing variables or by defining new variables with clear boundaries. The system can determine how the new input interacts with the existing structure because the components of that structure are well-defined. When boundaries are unstable, integration becomes inconsistent. New inputs may be forced into existing terms that do not fully represent them, or they may create overlapping variables that fragment the model. This reduces coherence and increases the likelihood of contradiction.

Concept stability also determines scalability. As problems increase in complexity, the system must manage a larger number of variables and relationships. Stable definitions allow these elements to be combined without losing clarity. Each variable retains its identity, and relationships can be extended without redefining the components involved. When definitions are unstable, complexity leads to collapse. The system cannot maintain clear distinctions between variables, and relationships become increasingly ambiguous. This limits the system's ability to handle more complex scenarios.

Maintaining boundaries requires explicit definition and consistent application. Variables must be defined in a way that captures their structure without unnecessary expansion. Once defined, those boundaries must remain fixed unless a change is made deliberately and applied consistently across the model. When a definition changes, the system must update all relationships that depend on it to maintain continuity. This ensures that the model remains coherent and that reasoning processes operate on stable elements.

When definitions function as boundaries, the system gains control over its representations. It can track variables across transformations, maintain relationships without distortion, and identify errors with precision. Concepts become reliable components within the architecture rather than shifting labels that introduce ambiguity. This stability allows the system to build more complex models without losing alignment, because each element within the model retains its identity and interacts with others in a defined and traceable way.

Variable Clarity

A thinking system can only preserve relationships if the variables it operates on remain stable across time and context. Variable clarity defines what a term refers to, where its boundaries begin and end, and how it differs from adjacent variables. This clarity allows the system to track a variable as it moves through different stages of reasoning without losing its identity. When clarity is maintained, each transformation operates on the same object, and the relationships built on that object remain consistent. When clarity degrades, the system begins to operate on shifting representations, and the output reflects that instability rather than the structure of the problem.

Semantic drift occurs when a variable changes meaning without explicit recognition. The label remains constant, but the underlying structure it represents shifts as it is used in different contexts. This shift may be gradual, with small expansions or contractions of scope that accumulate over time. The system continues to treat the variable as stable because the term has not changed, but the content of the variable no longer matches its original definition. This introduces hidden inconsistency. Relationships that were valid under the initial definition no longer apply, but the system continues to use them as if they do.

Clarity prevents this by enforcing fixed boundaries. A variable must be defined in a way that excludes what it is not, not just includes what it is. This exclusion is what maintains separation between variables and allows the system to assign relationships precisely. If a variable expands to include additional elements without being redefined, it begins to overlap with other variables. The system loses the ability to distinguish which component is responsible for a given effect. Relationships become generalized because the variable no longer corresponds to a specific structure.

As reasoning progresses, variable clarity supports continuity. Each step depends on the assumption that the variables being manipulated are the same ones that were defined at the start. If a variable is reinterpreted mid-process, the chain of reasoning breaks. The conclusion may still appear coherent, but it is no longer derived from the original structure. The system cannot trace how the output relates to the input because the elements have changed during the transformation. This loss of continuity undermines both accuracy and traceability.

Semantic drift also interferes with integration. When new information is introduced, the system must determine how it maps onto existing variables. If those variables are clearly defined, the mapping can be precise. The system can identify whether the new input fits within an existing boundary or requires the creation of a new variable. If the boundaries are ambiguous, the system may force the new input into an existing term that does not fully represent it. This creates overlap and inconsistency. Over time, the model becomes fragmented because variables no longer correspond to distinct structures.

Error detection depends on variable clarity. When a prediction fails, the system must isolate which part of the model produced the mismatch. If variables are stable, the system can identify whether the error originates from the definition of a variable or from the relationship applied to it. If variables have drifted, this isolation is not possible. The system cannot determine whether the failure is due to incorrect relationships or to changes in what the variables represent. Correction becomes inefficient because it targets multiple components without resolving the underlying issue.

Compression accelerates drift. When complex variables are reduced to simplified terms, internal distinctions are removed. The term begins to represent a broader set of elements, each with potentially different behaviors. The system gains efficiency, but it loses the ability to differentiate between those elements. As the term is used across contexts, its meaning expands further, incorporating additional associations. The variable becomes a container for loosely related concepts rather than a defined structure. This increases the likelihood of applying relationships that do not hold for all elements within the variable.

Maintaining variable clarity requires active constraint. Definitions must be explicit, and their boundaries must be preserved as the variable is used. When a change in meaning is necessary, it must be treated as a redefinition rather than an implicit shift. This involves updating the relationships that depend on the variable to reflect the new structure. Without this process, the system accumulates hidden inconsistencies that degrade accuracy over time.

Clarity also supports scalability. As the number of variables increases, the system must manage more relationships without losing track of individual components. Stable definitions allow variables to be combined and recombined without ambiguity. Each element retains its identity, and interactions can be extended to more complex systems without redefining the components involved. When clarity is absent, increasing complexity amplifies drift. Variables overlap, relationships become indistinct, and the system's ability to maintain alignment declines.

Preventing semantic drift is not a one-time correction. It is an ongoing requirement for maintaining a functional model. The system must continuously ensure that variables retain their defined structure and that any changes are explicit and consistently applied. When this condition is met, reasoning operates on stable elements, relationships remain valid across contexts, and outputs reflect the structure of the problem rather than the instability of the representations used to describe it.

Ambiguity as Structural Failure

A thinking system relies on language to construct and manipulate its internal model. Words define variables, encode relationships, and carry those relationships across each stage of reasoning. When language is precise, the system operates on stable representations that preserve structure. When language is ambiguous, the system loses that stability at the point of definition. The failure is not superficial. It alters the architecture of the model by introducing uncertainty into what the variables are and how they interact.

Ambiguity begins when a term does not map to a single, clearly bounded structure. The same word may refer to multiple underlying concepts, or its boundaries may be undefined, allowing it to expand or contract depending on context. The system continues to use the term as if it were stable, but each use may reference a different structure. This creates hidden variation within the model. Relationships that appear consistent at the level of language are applied to different underlying variables, producing outputs that do not preserve the intended interactions.

As reasoning progresses, this instability propagates. Each step in the process depends on the assumption that variables remain constant as they are transformed. When a variable shifts meaning between steps, the transformation no longer operates on the same object. The output may follow from the immediate step, but it does not follow from the original input. The system loses continuity. It cannot maintain a coherent pathway from input to output because the elements within that pathway are not fixed.

Ambiguity also distorts relationships. If the variables involved in a relationship are not clearly defined, the system cannot specify how they interact. It may describe the interaction in general terms, but those terms do not capture the conditions, direction, or magnitude of the relationship. This leads to overgeneralization. The system applies the same relationship across contexts where it does not hold because the lack of definition prevents it from identifying the boundaries within which the relationship is valid.

Error detection depends on the ability to isolate discrepancies within the model. When language is precise, a mismatch between prediction and outcome can be traced to a specific variable or relationship. The system can identify where the structure failed and adjust that component. When language is ambiguous, this isolation is not possible. The system cannot determine whether the error originates from the definition of a variable, the relationship applied to it, or a shift in meaning that occurred during reasoning. Correction becomes broad and inefficient, often failing to address the source of the problem.

Ambiguity is reinforced by compression and convenience. Simplified language reduces cognitive load, allowing the system to process information more quickly. However, this simplification removes detail that may be necessary to preserve structure. Terms become placeholders for complex sets of variables and interactions without exposing their internal composition. As these terms are reused across contexts, their meanings expand and overlap. The system gains efficiency but loses the ability to differentiate between distinct structures.

The effect becomes more pronounced as complexity increases. In simple scenarios, ambiguity may not produce visible errors because the number of variables and relationships is limited. As the system attempts to handle more complex problems, the lack of precise definitions prevents it from maintaining clear distinctions. Variables overlap, relationships become indistinct, and the model loses coherence. The system may still generate outputs, but those outputs are based on approximations rather than on defined interactions.

Ambiguity also allows contradictions to persist. When terms are not clearly defined, conflicting statements can coexist because the system interprets the same word differently in each context. This prevents the model from recognizing inconsistency. The system appears coherent because each statement is locally valid under its interpretation, but the overall structure contains incompatible elements that have not been reconciled.

Restoring structural integrity requires eliminating ambiguity at the level of representation. Variables must be defined with boundaries that prevent overlap, and those definitions must be applied consistently. Relationships must be expressed in a way that specifies how variables interact under defined conditions. As reasoning progresses, the system must ensure that terms retain their meaning and that any change in definition is explicit and propagated through the model.

When ambiguity is removed, the system regains the ability to preserve structure across transformations. Variables remain stable, relationships remain valid, and outputs can be traced back to their origin. Reasoning becomes a process of manipulating defined elements rather than navigating shifting representations. This restores alignment because the model once again reflects the structure it is intended to represent, rather than the instability introduced by unclear language.

Chapter 7

Inference Mechanics

A thinking system produces reliable conclusions only when it can transform inputs into outputs while preserving the relationships that define the problem. Inference is the mechanism that performs this transformation. It is not the act of reaching a conclusion. It is the sequence of operations that carries structure from the input through intermediate representations to the output without introducing distortion. Each step in this sequence must operate on defined variables, maintain their boundaries, and apply relationships that are consistent with both the model and the environment. When this sequence is intact, conclusions are not guessed or retrieved. They are constructed.

Inference begins with decomposition. An input is not processed as a whole. It is separated into variables that can be individually defined and tracked. This step determines the resolution of the model. If variables are too broad, important distinctions are lost. If they are too fragmented, relationships become difficult to manage. The system must identify components that capture the structure of the input without introducing unnecessary complexity. These components become the units on which all subsequent operations depend.

Once variables are defined, relationships between them must be established. These relationships encode how changes in one variable affect another under specific conditions. They are not descriptive. They are operational. The system uses them to generate expectations about how the model will behave when variables are manipulated. At this stage, the structure of the problem is represented internally. The model does not yet produce an output, but it defines the constraints that any valid output must satisfy.

Transformation occurs through the application of these relationships. The system modifies variables according to defined interactions, producing intermediate states that move the model toward a conclusion. Each transformation must preserve continuity. The variables at each stage must be traceable to their previous state, and the relationships applied must be consistent with those defined earlier. This creates a chain of states, each one derived from the last through operations that maintain structural integrity.

Validation is embedded within the sequence. At each stage, the system must ensure that the transformation has not introduced inconsistency. This does not require external feedback at every step, but it requires internal checks that confirm the relationships are being applied correctly. If a mismatch is detected, the system must halt or adjust before proceeding. This prevents errors from propagating through the sequence and affecting the final output.

As the system approaches a conclusion, the final state of the variables represents the output. This output is not independent of the process that produced it. It is the end point of a chain that has preserved relationships from the input. Because the pathway is explicit, the system can trace the output back through each transformation to verify its validity or to identify where an error may have occurred. This traceability is what allows inference to support correction as well as construction.

Inference differs from associative or heuristic processes in its reliance on explicit structure. Association moves between linked concepts without maintaining defined relationships. Heuristics compress sequences into shortcuts that bypass intermediate steps. Both can produce outputs quickly, but they do not preserve the pathway required for traceability and correction. Inference maintains that pathway. It operates more slowly, but it ensures that each output is anchored to the structure of the input.

The effectiveness of inference depends on the stability of the variables and relationships it operates on. If definitions are ambiguous or if relationships are underdefined, the sequence cannot maintain continuity. Transformations will operate on shifting elements, and the output will not correspond to the intended structure. Inference does not correct for instability at the level of representation. It requires that stability to function.

Environmental conditions influence how often inference is used. Under time pressure or high input volume, the system may default to faster processes that bypass structured transformation. Over time, this reduces the system's tendency to engage inference even when it is necessary. The capacity remains, but it is not activated consistently. This leads to a system that can perform structured reasoning but does not rely on it as its primary mechanism.

Maintaining inference as the dominant process requires preserving its sequence. Inputs must be decomposed into stable variables, relationships must be explicitly defined, transformations must preserve continuity, and validation must occur at each stage. When these conditions are met, inference produces outputs that are both accurate and traceable. The system does not depend on external correction to maintain alignment because its internal process enforces the preservation of structure from input to output.

Inference mechanics define how thinking operates at the structural level. They determine whether the system constructs conclusions that correspond to reality or generates outputs that are internally coherent but externally misaligned. When the mechanism is intact, accuracy emerges from the process itself. When it is degraded, the system may still produce answers, but those answers are no longer constrained by the relationships that define what is true.

Premise → Inference → Conclusion

A reasoning system produces a valid conclusion only when it preserves structure across the entire chain from premise to output. The premise defines the initial state of the model. It establishes the variables, their boundaries, and the relationships that are assumed to hold. The inference process transforms that initial state through a sequence of operations that must maintain those relationships without introducing distortion. The conclusion is the final state of the system after those transformations have been applied. If any part of this chain fails, the conclusion no longer reflects the structure defined by the premise.

The premise is not a statement in isolation. It is a structured input that encodes conditions about the system being modeled. Each variable within the premise must be clearly defined, and each relationship must specify how those variables interact. If the premise contains ambiguity, the system begins with unstable components. This instability cannot be corrected later in the chain because every transformation depends on the initial definitions. The quality of the conclusion is constrained by the integrity of the premise. An imprecise premise produces a model that cannot support precise reasoning.

Inference operates as a controlled transformation of the premise. The system applies defined relationships to the variables, generating intermediate states that move the model toward an output. Each step must preserve continuity. Variables must retain their identity, and relationships must be applied under the conditions in which they are valid. If a variable shifts meaning during this process or if a relationship is applied outside its defined scope, the transformation introduces error. This error propagates forward because each subsequent step builds on the previous state.

The sequence of transformations forms a pathway that connects the premise to the conclusion. This pathway must remain traceable. Each intermediate state should be derivable from the one before it through operations that are consistent with the model. Traceability allows the system to verify the conclusion by retracing the steps taken. If the pathway cannot be reconstructed, the system cannot determine whether the conclusion follows from the premise or from unintended changes introduced during processing.

The conclusion represents the final configuration of the variables after all transformations have been applied. It is not independent of the process. It is the end point of the chain. A valid conclusion is one that can be derived from the premise through a sequence of transformations that preserve structure. If the conclusion introduces elements that were not present in the premise or inferred through valid relationships, it is not connected to the original model. It may appear plausible, but it is not the result of the defined process.

Failure within the chain occurs in distinct ways. The premise may be unstable, with variables that lack clear boundaries or relationships that are not specified. In this case, the system begins with an undefined model. Inference may be incomplete or distorted, with steps that skip necessary transformations or apply relationships inconsistently. This breaks continuity. The conclusion may be detached, presenting an output that does not follow from the transformations applied. Each type of failure disrupts the alignment between the initial conditions and the final result.

Time pressure and cognitive load increase the likelihood of chain compression. The system reduces the number of explicit steps by collapsing multiple transformations into a single operation. This increases speed but removes visibility into how the conclusion was reached. Without intermediate states, the system cannot verify whether each transformation preserved structure. Errors become difficult to detect because the pathway is no longer explicit.

Associative processes bypass the chain entirely. Instead of transforming the premise through defined relationships, the system retrieves a conclusion based on similarity or familiarity. The output may align with past patterns, but it is not derived from the current premise. This breaks the connection between input and output. The system produces a result without constructing the pathway that would justify it.

Maintaining the full chain requires explicit control over each stage. The premise must be defined with clear variables and relationships. Inference must proceed through steps that preserve those definitions and apply relationships under appropriate conditions. The conclusion must emerge from that sequence without introducing elements that were not part of the model. When these conditions are met, the system produces outputs that are structurally linked to their inputs.

The full chain ensures that reasoning remains anchored to reality. The premise encodes the structure of the environment, inference preserves that structure through transformation, and the conclusion reflects the resulting state of the system. When the chain is intact, accuracy is not an isolated property of the output. It is a consequence of the process that produced it.

Valid vs Invalid Transitions

A reasoning system does not fail at the level of conclusions. It fails at the level of transitions. Each step between states either preserves the structure defined by the model or alters it in a way that breaks continuity. A valid transition carries variables forward without changing their identity and applies relationships within the conditions that define them. An invalid transition introduces a change that is not accounted for in the model. This change may be subtle, but once it occurs, every subsequent step operates on a distorted state.

A transition begins with a defined state of variables and relationships. The system applies an operation that modifies one or more variables according to those relationships. For the transition to be valid, the operation must be consistent with the structure of the model. The variables must retain their boundaries, and the relationship used must match the conditions under which it is defined. If either of these conditions is violated, the transition produces a new state that is not structurally equivalent to the one expected.

Invalid transitions often occur when variables shift during processing. A term may refer to a specific component at one stage and a broader category at the next. The label remains constant, but the underlying structure changes. The system applies a relationship that was valid for the original definition to a modified variable. This creates a mismatch between the operation and the object it is applied to. The resulting state appears coherent, but it is built on an inconsistency that was introduced at the point of transition.

Another source of invalid transitions is the misapplication of relationships. A relationship defines how variables interact under specific conditions. When the system applies that relationship outside those conditions, the transformation no longer reflects the behavior of the model. The variables may remain stable, but the interaction between them is no longer accurate. This produces a state that deviates from what the model would predict if the relationship were applied correctly.

Tracking logical movement requires maintaining visibility into each transition. The system must be able to identify the variables involved, the relationship applied, and the resulting change in state. This visibility allows the system to verify that each step preserves structure. When transitions are compressed or skipped, this verification is lost. The system moves from one state to another without an explicit pathway, making it difficult to detect where an error may have been introduced.

Valid transitions form a continuous chain. Each state is derived from the previous one through operations that maintain consistency with the model. This continuity allows the system to trace the pathway from the initial premise to the final conclusion. If a mismatch is detected at the conclusion, the system can move backward through the chain to locate the transition where the structure was first altered. This enables targeted correction rather than broad adjustments.

Invalid transitions break this continuity. Once a transition introduces an unaccounted change, the subsequent states are no longer connected to the original model in a consistent way. The system may continue to apply valid operations to the new state, but those operations are now acting on a distorted representation. The error compounds because each step builds on the altered state rather than on the original structure.

Heuristic and associative processes increase the frequency of invalid transitions. These processes prioritize speed by reducing the number of explicit steps. Relationships are applied in generalized form, and variables are treated as interchangeable within broad categories. This removes the constraints that ensure transitions remain valid. The system produces outputs quickly, but it does so by bypassing the checks that would preserve structural integrity.

Maintaining valid transitions requires explicit control over both variables and relationships. Variables must remain stable across steps, and relationships must be applied only within their defined scope.

Each transition must be represented as a discrete operation that can be inspected and verified. This does not require slowing the system unnecessarily, but it requires preserving enough detail to ensure that each step maintains alignment with the model.

Logical movement is the accumulation of these transitions. It is not defined by the final answer but by the pathway that leads to it. When transitions are valid, the pathway preserves the structure of the problem, and the conclusion reflects that structure. When transitions are invalid, the pathway diverges, and the conclusion no longer corresponds to the original model. Accuracy is therefore a function of maintaining valid transitions throughout the sequence, not of selecting a plausible endpoint.

Error Localization

A reasoning system does not correct itself by evaluating the conclusion in isolation. It corrects itself by locating the exact point in the chain where structure was first altered. Error localization is the process of tracing a mismatch back through the sequence of transitions to identify the earliest deviation from the defined model. This requires that each step in the reasoning chain remains explicit, with variables, relationships, and transformations preserved in a way that can be inspected. Without this visibility, the system cannot isolate the source of the error and is forced to adjust multiple components without knowing which one caused the failure.

The process begins with detection. A mismatch appears when the output of the system does not align with expected behavior or with external feedback. This mismatch signals that somewhere in the chain, a transition did not preserve structure. The system must then move backward through the sequence of states, examining each transition in reverse order. At each step, it compares the expected transformation, based on the defined relationships, with the actual transformation that occurred. The goal is to find the first point where these diverge.

Localization depends on stable variables. If the variables involved in each step retain their identity, the system can track them across transitions and determine whether their state changed in a way that is consistent with the model. If variables have drifted or been redefined during processing, the system cannot perform this comparison accurately. It may identify discrepancies, but it cannot determine whether they originate from incorrect transformations or from changes in what the variables represent. This prevents precise localization.

Relationships must also remain defined. Each transition applies a relationship under specific conditions. When tracing an error, the system must verify that the relationship used at each step matches the conditions present in the variables at that stage. If a relationship was applied outside its valid scope, the transformation at that step becomes the point of failure. If relationships are loosely defined, the system cannot determine whether they were applied correctly, and the search for the error becomes diffuse.

The earliest invalid transition is the critical point. Later steps may appear incorrect because they build on a distorted state, but correcting those steps does not resolve the underlying issue. The system must identify the first deviation, because that is where the model diverged from its defined structure. Once this point is located, the system can correct the transition by restoring the proper variable definition or applying the correct relationship. Subsequent steps can then be recalculated from this corrected state.

Compression interferes with localization. When multiple transitions are collapsed into a single step, the internal operations are no longer visible. The system can detect that an error exists within that compressed segment, but it cannot isolate which part of the transformation caused it. This forces the system to expand the segment or to reconstruct intermediate states in order to regain visibility. Without this reconstruction, correction remains imprecise.

Associative reasoning eliminates the pathway required for localization. When a conclusion is produced through pattern matching rather than through explicit transformation, there are no intermediate states to inspect. The system cannot trace how the output was derived from the input because the process bypassed structured inference. In this case, error localization is not possible within the reasoning chain itself. The system must reconstruct a structured pathway after the fact to identify where alignment would have failed.

Effective localization requires that the system maintain a continuous record of transitions. Each step must be defined in terms of the variables involved, the relationship applied, and the resulting change in state. This record does not need to be externalized in full detail, but it must be preserved internally in a way that allows backward traversal. When a mismatch occurs, the system can then move through this record, isolating the point at which the transformation no longer matches the model.

Correction follows localization. Once the first invalid transition is identified, the system adjusts the variable definition or relationship at that point and then propagates the correction forward. This restores continuity between the premise and the conclusion. Without localization, correction becomes broad and inefficient, often addressing symptoms rather than the cause.

Error localization maintains alignment over time. It allows the system to refine its model by identifying and correcting specific points of failure rather than making generalized adjustments. This preserves the integrity of the reasoning process because each correction is tied to a defined component within the architecture. The system does not rely on guesswork or external correction alone. It uses its internal structure to identify where it diverged and to restore that structure at the exact point of breakdown.

Chapter 8

Constraints and Systems

A system does not behave according to what it intends to do. It behaves according to what its constraints allow. Every process, whether biological, mechanical, or cognitive, operates within boundaries that define what states are possible and how transitions between those states can occur. These constraints are not external limitations layered on top of a system. They are embedded within its structure. They determine capacity, speed, precision, and stability. When outcomes diverge from expectation, the cause is not a failure of effort or input. It is a mismatch between the demands placed on the system and the constraints that govern its operation.

Constraints exist at multiple levels. At the lowest level, structure defines what the system is physically capable of doing. Components have properties that limit how they can interact. In biological systems, membrane composition determines permeability, receptor configuration determines signaling sensitivity, and enzyme structure determines reaction rates. These are not adjustable through intention. They define the operational space of the system. At higher levels, constraints emerge from organization. The arrangement of components determines how signals propagate, how resources are allocated, and how feedback is processed. These organizational constraints shape behavior even when the underlying components remain unchanged.

Throughput is one of the primary expressions of constraint. A system can only process a certain volume of input within a given time frame.

When input exceeds this capacity, the system does not scale linearly. It degrades. Steps are skipped, precision decreases, and outputs become less aligned with the structure of the input. This degradation is not random. It follows directly from the system attempting to operate beyond its defined limits. In cognitive systems, increased input volume leads to compression of reasoning steps. In metabolic systems, excess substrate leads to incomplete processing and accumulation of intermediates. The pattern is consistent because the underlying principle is the same.

Time functions as a constraint on feedback. Systems rely on feedback to adjust their internal state based on the results of their actions. When feedback is immediate, the system can correct errors at the point of occurrence. When feedback is delayed, the system continues to operate on an outdated model. This introduces drift. Actions are taken based on assumptions that no longer reflect current conditions. The longer the delay, the greater the divergence between the system's internal state and the environment it is interacting with. Correction becomes more difficult because the system must reconcile multiple layers of accumulated error.

Energy is another defining constraint. Every transformation requires resources. In biological systems, energy availability determines whether processes can proceed, how quickly they occur, and how accurately they are executed. When energy is limited, the system prioritizes essential functions and reduces investment in processes that require precision. This tradeoff affects quality. Reactions may still occur, but they occur under conditions that increase the likelihood of error or incomplete completion. In cognitive systems, limited energy manifests as reduced capacity for structured reasoning, with a shift toward faster, less precise processes.

Constraints also define tradeoffs. A system cannot maximize all variables simultaneously. Increasing speed often reduces accuracy. Expanding capacity may reduce stability. Enhancing sensitivity may increase susceptibility to noise. These tradeoffs are not optional. They are built into the structure of the system. Understanding them allows the system to allocate resources in a way that aligns with its objectives. Ignoring them leads to attempts to achieve incompatible outcomes, resulting in instability or failure.

Systems maintain stability through feedback loops that operate within these constraints. Feedback allows the system to detect deviations from its desired state and to adjust accordingly. For feedback to function, the system must be able to detect changes, process that information, and implement a response. Each of these steps is constrained. Detection depends on sensor resolution, processing depends on computational capacity, and response depends on the ability to modify internal variables. If any part of this loop is limited, the system's ability to maintain alignment is reduced.

When constraints are exceeded or ignored, systems do not fail gradually in a visible way. They accumulate internal strain until a threshold is reached, after which failure appears sudden. This apparent suddenness is a result of hidden accumulation. The system has been operating outside its optimal range, and small deviations have compounded over time. Once the accumulated error surpasses the system's ability to compensate, the output shifts abruptly. The failure is structural, not event-driven.

Understanding a system requires identifying its constraints before analyzing its behavior. Behavior is the result of how the system operates within those boundaries. Attempts to modify outcomes without addressing constraints are limited because they do not change the conditions that produce those outcomes. Adjusting inputs may produce temporary changes, but the system will return to behavior that is consistent with its structure.

Control emerges from alignment with constraints. When the system operates within its defined limits, processes remain stable, feedback functions effectively, and outputs reflect the structure of the model. When demands exceed those limits, the system shifts into states that prioritize survival over precision, leading to degraded performance. This shift is not a failure of the system. It is the system operating according to its design under different conditions.

Constraints define what a system can do, how it does it, and how it fails. They are the framework within which all processes occur. Understanding them allows the system to predict behavior, identify points of failure, and adjust operations in a way that maintains alignment. Without this understanding, analysis focuses on outputs without recognizing the structure that produces them, and correction remains disconnected from the mechanisms that determine what is possible.

Logic as Constraint System

Logic does not generate conclusions by expanding possibility. It restricts possibility. It defines a bounded space of outcomes that can exist given a set of premises and relationships, and it eliminates everything outside that space. The function of logic is therefore not creative in the sense of producing new options. It is reductive. It removes invalid states until only those that preserve the structure of the model remain. What appears as a conclusion is the result of this constraint process applied across a sequence of valid transitions.

A premise establishes the initial constraints. It defines the variables, their boundaries, and the relationships that govern how those variables can change. These constraints are not descriptive statements. They are conditions that limit what transformations are allowed. Once defined, they form the permissible state space of the system. Any conclusion must exist within this space. If an output requires violating one of these constraints, it is not a valid extension of the premise, regardless of how plausible it appears.

Inference operates by applying constraints step by step. Each transformation reduces the number of possible states by enforcing relationships that must hold. This reduction is cumulative. With each valid transition, the system eliminates configurations that do not satisfy the conditions imposed by the model. The pathway from premise to conclusion is therefore a narrowing process. It moves from a broader set of possible states to a smaller set that remains consistent with all applied constraints.

Invalid reasoning introduces states that lie outside this constrained space. This occurs when a relationship is applied beyond its defined conditions or when a variable is altered without preserving its boundaries. The system then operates on a configuration that is not permitted by the original model. Subsequent steps may be internally consistent with this altered state, but they no longer correspond to the constraints defined by the premise. The conclusion reflects the modified system rather than the one originally specified.

Constraint integrity determines whether logic can function as intended. Variables must remain stable, and relationships must be applied only within their valid scope. If constraints are ambiguous, the system cannot enforce them. It may allow multiple interpretations of the same condition, effectively expanding the permissible state space beyond what was intended. This weakens the filtering process. Invalid states are no longer excluded, and the system can arrive at conclusions that do not preserve the structure of the premise.

Logical consistency is not sufficient on its own. A system can produce conclusions that are internally consistent while still violating external constraints. This occurs when the internal model does not accurately represent the conditions it is meant to describe. Logic ensures that transformations within the model are valid, but it does not guarantee that the model itself is aligned with reality. Constraint accuracy must therefore exist at both levels. Internal constraints must be applied correctly, and those constraints must correspond to actual conditions.

As complexity increases, the role of constraints becomes more critical. The number of possible states grows rapidly as more variables and relationships are introduced. Without a mechanism to limit this space, the system cannot maintain control over the reasoning process. Logic provides that mechanism by enforcing conditions that eliminate invalid configurations at each step. This prevents the system from exploring paths that do not lead to valid conclusions.

Compression and heuristic processing weaken constraint enforcement. When multiple steps are collapsed, the intermediate constraints that would normally restrict the state space are not explicitly applied. The system moves from premise to conclusion without performing the full sequence of reductions. This increases the likelihood of including states that should have been excluded. The output may still align with expectations in simple cases, but as complexity increases, the absence of constraint enforcement leads to divergence.

Maintaining logic as a constraint system requires explicit representation of both variables and relationships. Each step in the reasoning process must apply the constraints that define the model. This ensures that the state space is progressively reduced in a controlled manner. The conclusion then emerges as the remaining state or set of states that satisfy all conditions.

The value of logic lies in this restriction. By limiting what is possible, it ensures that conclusions are not selected based on familiarity, coherence, or preference. They are derived from the structure of the system. When constraints are enforced consistently, the system cannot produce outputs that violate its own definitions. This does not guarantee that the model is correct, but it guarantees that the reasoning process remains aligned with the model that has been defined.

Variables and Interactions

A system is defined by its variables and the interactions that connect them. Variables represent discrete components with boundaries that determine what is included and what is excluded. Interactions define how changes in one variable propagate through the system and alter the state of others. Without clearly defined variables, interactions cannot be specified. Without defined interactions, variables remain isolated and cannot produce behavior. The structure of the system emerges from the mapping between these two elements.

A variable must correspond to a specific structure or process. It cannot function as a general label that covers multiple distinct components unless those components behave identically under all relevant conditions. When a variable contains internal variation, the system loses resolution. Interactions applied to that variable become approximations because they cannot account for differences between the elements it represents. This leads to outputs that reflect averaged behavior rather than the actual response of any specific component.

Interactions encode direction and condition. They specify how a change in one variable affects another and under what circumstances that effect occurs. This includes magnitude, timing, and dependency. An interaction is not simply a connection. It defines the rules of transformation between variables. If those rules are not specified, the system cannot predict how a change will propagate. It can describe associations, but it cannot generate controlled transformations that preserve structure.

Mapping relationships requires identifying both direct and indirect interactions. A direct interaction occurs when a change in one variable produces an immediate change in another through a defined mechanism. An indirect interaction occurs when the effect is mediated through one or more intermediate variables. The system must distinguish between these types because they differ in timing, magnitude, and susceptibility to modification. Treating indirect interactions as direct compresses the pathway and removes the intermediate structure that determines how the effect unfolds.

The configuration of interactions determines system behavior. Variables do not act independently. Their effects depend on the network they are part of. A change in one variable may produce different outcomes depending on the state of other variables and the pathways through which the interaction occurs. This context dependence is a result of the structure of the interaction network. The same variable can produce different outputs because it is embedded in a system where multiple pathways converge and diverge.

Nonlinear interactions arise when the effect of a change in one variable depends on the current state of another. In these cases, the relationship cannot be represented as a fixed proportional change. The system must account for thresholds, saturation points, and feedback loops that alter how variables influence each other. These features are not secondary details. They define how the system transitions between states and how it responds to perturbations.

Feedback loops are a specific class of interaction where the output of a process influences its own input. Positive feedback amplifies changes, pushing the system further in the direction of the initial shift. Negative feedback counteracts changes, stabilizing the system around a set point. The presence and strength of these loops determine whether the system remains stable, oscillates, or transitions into a different state. Mapping these loops requires identifying not only the variables involved but also the direction and timing of the feedback.

Accurate mapping requires maintaining separation between variables. Overlapping definitions create ambiguity in interactions. If two variables share components, the system cannot determine which variable is responsible for a given effect. This leads to redundant or conflicting interactions that reduce clarity. Each variable must represent a distinct element, and interactions must be defined between those elements without overlap.

As complexity increases, the number of variables and interactions grows. The system must maintain organization to prevent collapse into undifferentiated connections. This involves grouping variables into subsystems and defining interactions at multiple levels. Lower-level interactions define local behavior, while higher-level interactions define how subsystems influence each other. This hierarchical structure allows the system to scale without losing clarity.

Mapping relationships is not a static process. As new information is introduced, variables may need to be refined, and interactions may need to be updated. This requires maintaining flexibility without sacrificing stability. Changes must be explicit and propagated through the network to preserve consistency. If updates are applied locally without adjusting related interactions, the system accumulates inconsistencies that degrade accuracy.

When variables are clearly defined and interactions are precisely mapped, the system can generate predictions that reflect its structure. Changes in input produce changes in output that can be traced through the network of relationships. This traceability allows the system to verify its behavior and to identify where deviations occur. Without this mapping, the system operates on disconnected elements, and outputs become dependent on approximation rather than on defined interactions.

Multi-Variable Complexity

A system with a single variable can be approximated. A system with many variables cannot be compressed without losing structure. As the number of variables increases, the number of possible interactions expands in a non-linear way. Each additional variable does not add a single new pathway. It introduces a set of interactions with every existing variable, along with conditional dependencies that alter how those interactions behave under different states. The system moves from a simple mapping to a network where outcomes depend on configurations rather than on isolated inputs.

Heuristics operate by collapsing this network into simplified patterns. They replace explicit relationships with generalized rules that approximate common outcomes. This works when the system is low-dimensional and the interactions are relatively stable. The heuristic captures enough of the structure to produce acceptable results. As dimensionality increases, this compression removes too much information. The heuristic no longer represents the system. It represents a reduced model that cannot account for the variability introduced by additional variables.

The failure emerges through interaction density. When variables interact in pairs, the system must account for the conditions under which each interaction is active and how the magnitude of one effect depends on the state of another variable. When interactions extend across three or more variables, dependencies become conditional on combinations of states. A change in one variable may produce different outcomes depending on the configuration of several others. Heuristics cannot encode these conditional layers. They apply the same rule across contexts that require different responses.

Nonlinearity amplifies this problem. In multi-variable systems, relationships are rarely proportional. Effects may increase up to a threshold and then plateau, reverse, or trigger secondary pathways. The response curve depends on the current state of the system, not just on the magnitude of the input. Heuristics treat relationships as fixed patterns. They do not adjust based on state because they do not track the variables required to determine that state. This leads to systematic error when the system moves outside the conditions under which the heuristic was formed.

State dependence further increases complexity. The system's history influences its current behavior. Variables may carry forward effects from prior states, altering how they respond to new inputs. This introduces temporal layering. The same input applied at different times produces different outputs because the underlying configuration has changed. Heuristics do not track state history in a structured way. They operate on the current input without reconstructing the pathway that led to the present configuration.

Feedback loops create additional failure points. When outputs feed back into inputs, the system evolves over time based on its own behavior. Positive feedback can amplify small differences into large divergences. Negative feedback can stabilize the system within a narrow range. The presence of these loops means that a small error introduced by a heuristic can propagate and expand. Because the heuristic does not model the loop explicitly, it cannot predict how that error will evolve across iterations.

As the system scales, interactions begin to overlap. Variables influence the same downstream components through different pathways. The combined effect depends on how these pathways converge. Heuristics treat these influences independently or merge them into a single simplified rule. This removes the ability to distinguish which pathway is responsible for a given outcome and how their interactions modify the result. The system loses resolution at the point where it is most needed.

Combinatorial growth makes exhaustive evaluation impractical. The number of possible states increases rapidly with each additional variable. A structured system manages this by applying constraints that eliminate invalid states and by tracking only the pathways that remain consistent with those constraints. Heuristics bypass this process. They do not reduce the state space through controlled elimination. They select a likely outcome based on pattern similarity. As the number of variables increases, the distance between the heuristic's pattern and the actual state of the system grows, reducing accuracy.

Error accumulation becomes unavoidable. Each heuristic approximation introduces a small deviation from the system's true behavior. In low-dimensional systems, these deviations may remain within acceptable bounds. In high-dimensional systems, deviations interact. An error in one variable alters the conditions under which other variables operate, producing additional errors that compound over time. The system diverges from the structure it is meant to represent.

Maintaining accuracy at scale requires preserving the architecture of the system. Variables must be tracked individually, interactions must be defined with their conditions, and transformations must be applied in a way that accounts for state dependence and feedback. This does not eliminate complexity, but it allows the system to manage it by constraining possible states and maintaining traceability.

Heuristics fail at scale because they replace structure with approximation. They remove the relationships that define how variables interact and substitute patterns that only hold under limited conditions. As complexity increases, those conditions are rarely met. The system continues to produce outputs, but those outputs are no longer anchored to the underlying architecture. Accuracy is lost not because the system lacks information, but because it no longer preserves the structure required to use that information correctly.

PART III

DISTORTED THINKING SYSTEMS

Chapter 9

Cognitive Failures

A cognitive system fails when it can no longer preserve alignment between its internal model and the environment it is attempting to represent. This failure does not originate at the level of conclusions. It emerges from structural degradation within the system itself. Variables lose definition, relationships are applied outside their valid scope, and transitions no longer preserve continuity. The system continues to produce outputs, but those outputs are no longer constrained by the architecture that defines valid reasoning. What appears as error is the visible result of a deeper breakdown in how the system processes and maintains structure.

Failure often begins with variable instability. When definitions are not maintained, the system operates on elements that shift during processing. A variable may refer to one structure at the start of reasoning and a different structure by the time it is used in a later step. The label remains constant, masking the change. Relationships that were valid under the initial definition are applied to the altered variable, producing outputs that do not reflect the intended model. This instability propagates because each subsequent step builds on the distorted representation.

Relationship degradation follows. A system must apply interactions under the conditions that define them. When those conditions are ignored or simplified, relationships become generalized. The system treats context-dependent interactions as if they were universal. This removes the constraints that limit when and how variables influence each other. The result is a model that appears coherent internally but fails to produce accurate predictions when conditions change.

Transition breakdown is the next layer. Reasoning depends on a sequence of transformations that preserve structure from input to output. When transitions are skipped, compressed, or executed without verification, continuity is lost. The system moves between states without maintaining a clear pathway. This prevents traceability. When an error appears, the system cannot identify where the deviation occurred because the intermediate steps are not preserved.

Feedback failure accelerates the process. A system maintains alignment by comparing its outputs to external results and adjusting its internal model accordingly. When feedback is delayed, ignored, or misinterpreted, the system continues to operate on outdated assumptions. Errors accumulate because the system is not updating its structure in response to new information. The internal model diverges from the environment, and the gap widens over time.

Cognitive load and environmental pressure influence how these failures manifest. Under high input volume or time constraints, the system reduces the resolution of its processing. It compresses variables, simplifies relationships, and skips validation steps. This increases throughput but reduces accuracy. Over time, the system adapts to this mode of operation. Structured reasoning becomes less frequent, and the system relies more heavily on approximate processes that do not preserve architecture.

Associative processing replaces structured inference in this state. The system generates outputs based on similarity to past patterns rather than on transformations derived from the current input. This bypasses the chain that would normally connect premise to conclusion. The output may align with familiar scenarios, but it is not derived from the defined variables and relationships of the present problem. This creates a disconnect between input and output that cannot be corrected through traceability because the pathway was never constructed.

Confirmation bias emerges as a structural consequence of feedback failure. When the system does not incorporate corrective signals, it reinforces patterns that appear to produce consistent outputs. These patterns are treated as stable relationships even if they do not reflect the environment accurately. The system narrows its model around these patterns, reducing its ability to adapt when conditions change. This is not a preference for certain outcomes. It is a failure to update the structure that generates those outcomes.

Error accumulation produces drift. Small deviations introduced at the level of variables, relationships, or transitions compound over time. Each deviation alters the conditions under which subsequent operations occur. The system moves further from alignment with each step, even if individual errors appear minor. Eventually, the accumulated divergence reaches a point where outputs no longer correspond to the environment in a recognizable way. At this stage, failure appears abrupt, but it is the result of gradual structural degradation.

Recovery requires restoring the components that maintain alignment. Variables must be redefined with clear boundaries, relationships must be constrained to their valid conditions, and transitions must be made explicit and traceable. Feedback must be reintroduced in a way that allows the system to compare its outputs to external results and adjust accordingly. This process does not add new capabilities. It restores the architecture that allows the system to use its existing capabilities effectively.

Cognitive failures are not isolated mistakes. They are expressions of how the system is operating under its current constraints. When the architecture that preserves structure is degraded, the system cannot maintain alignment regardless of the information it has access to. When that architecture is intact, accuracy emerges from the process itself because each component functions within the conditions that define it.

Outcome Bias

A reasoning system cannot evaluate correctness from outcomes alone. An outcome is a terminal state. It contains no information about the sequence of transformations that produced it. When evaluation is based only on the result, the system removes the pathway that connects input to output. This breaks the link between structure and judgment. A correct outcome produced through invalid transitions appears acceptable, and an incorrect outcome produced through valid transitions appears flawed. The system loses the ability to distinguish between these cases because it is no longer inspecting the mechanism that generated the result.

Process defines whether a conclusion is valid. Each step in the reasoning chain must preserve variable identity, apply relationships within defined conditions, and maintain continuity from premise to conclusion. When this structure is intact, the conclusion is constrained by the model. When the structure is broken, the conclusion is unconstrained, even if it happens to align with the correct answer. Outcome bias replaces this structural evaluation with a binary check on the final state. The system asks whether the result matches an expected value, not whether the pathway that produced it was valid.

This creates false reinforcement. If an invalid process produces a correct outcome, the system registers the sequence as successful. The relationships and transitions used in that sequence are retained and reused, even though they do not preserve structure. Over time, these invalid patterns accumulate. The system begins to rely on transformations that work only under specific conditions or by coincidence. Accuracy appears stable in the short term, but the underlying model is degrading.

The inverse case produces false rejection. A valid process may produce an incorrect outcome when the premise is incomplete or when external conditions change. If evaluation is based only on the result, the system rejects the process that preserved structure and instead searches for an alternative that produces the expected output. This replaces a structurally sound pathway with one that may be less accurate but more likely to match the desired result under limited conditions. The system shifts away from processes that maintain alignment and toward those that optimize for outcome matching.

Outcome bias also prevents error localization. When a result is incorrect, the system must trace the reasoning chain to identify where the structure was altered. If the system evaluates only the outcome, it cannot determine whether the error originated from the premise, the relationships, or the transitions. Correction becomes broad. The system may adjust multiple components without isolating the source of the failure. This reduces efficiency and increases the likelihood of introducing additional errors.

The bias intensifies under conditions of delayed feedback. When the result of a decision is separated in time from the process that produced it, the system has limited visibility into the intermediate steps. The outcome becomes the only accessible signal. The system then relies more heavily on that signal for evaluation, further disconnecting judgment from process. Over time, the reasoning chain becomes compressed or bypassed because it is not being used for evaluation.

Complex systems amplify the effect. In multi-variable environments, the same outcome can be produced through different pathways. Some pathways preserve structure, while others introduce distortions that happen to cancel out under specific conditions. Outcome-based evaluation treats these pathways as equivalent because they produce the same result. The system cannot differentiate between a pathway that generalizes across conditions and one that only works within a narrow range.

Maintaining alignment requires shifting evaluation back to the process. Each step in the reasoning chain must be inspected to ensure that variables remain stable, relationships are applied correctly, and transitions preserve continuity. The outcome remains relevant, but it is used as a signal to trigger inspection rather than as the sole criterion for correctness. A correct outcome produced through invalid transitions is treated as a failure because it does not preserve the structure required for consistent performance. An incorrect outcome produced through valid transitions is treated as a model refinement problem rather than a reasoning failure.

This distinction preserves the integrity of the system. By evaluating the pathway instead of the endpoint, the system ensures that its internal operations remain aligned with the structure of the model. Outcomes then become a consequence of correct processing rather than the basis for determining it.

The Narrative Fallacy

A reasoning system fails when it substitutes sequence with story. Structure defines how variables interact under constraints to produce an outcome. A story defines a sequence of events that appears coherent when arranged in order. The two are not equivalent. Structure preserves causality through defined relationships. Narrative preserves coherence through interpretation. When narrative replaces structure, the system begins to treat a sequence that feels consistent as if it were a chain of valid transitions.

Narratives compress variables into roles. Instead of tracking distinct components with defined boundaries, the system assigns them simplified identities that fit within a storyline. These roles carry implicit assumptions about behavior. The system no longer evaluates how variables interact under specific conditions. It assumes that each role will behave according to the expectations embedded in the narrative. This removes the need to define relationships explicitly, but it also removes the constraints that ensure those relationships are valid.

Causality is replaced by temporal ordering. In a structured model, one variable affects another through a defined mechanism. The effect depends on the state of both variables and the conditions under which the interaction occurs. In a narrative, events are linked because they occur in sequence. The system interprets this sequence as causal even when no defined interaction exists. The presence of a temporal link is treated as sufficient explanation. This introduces relationships that are not grounded in the model.

Narratives also eliminate conditionality. Structured interactions specify when a relationship holds and when it does not. They define thresholds, dependencies, and context. A narrative presents a single pathway that appears to explain the outcome. It does not represent alternative states or conditions under which the sequence would change. The system loses the ability to evaluate how different configurations of variables would produce different results. It becomes locked into a single explanation that appears complete because it is internally coherent.

This compression interferes with error detection. When a narrative is used to explain an outcome, the system does not track individual transitions. It tracks the overall storyline. If the outcome is incorrect, the system cannot isolate which part of the sequence failed because the intermediate structure is not defined. The narrative can be adjusted by altering elements of the story, but this adjustment does not correspond to correcting specific variables or relationships. It changes the interpretation rather than the structure.

Narratives reinforce outcome bias. A story is often constructed after the outcome is known. The system selects elements that fit the result and arranges them into a coherent sequence. This creates the appearance that the outcome was predictable given the events described. The underlying reasoning process is not reconstructed. The system does not verify whether the sequence could have been generated through valid transitions from the original premise. It constructs a pathway that aligns with the outcome and treats it as if it were the actual process.

In multi-variable systems, the narrative fallacy becomes more pronounced. The number of possible interactions exceeds what can be represented in a simple sequence. The system reduces complexity by selecting a subset of variables that can be arranged into a linear story. This removes interactions that do not fit the narrative, even if they are necessary to explain the outcome. The resulting model is incomplete. It captures a simplified version of the system that cannot account for variations in conditions.

Narratives persist because they reduce cognitive load. They provide a compact representation that can be processed quickly. This efficiency comes at the cost of precision. The system trades the ability to track defined variables and interactions for the ability to generate a coherent explanation without explicit structure. As this mode of processing becomes dominant, the system loses the capacity to reconstruct the underlying architecture when needed.

Maintaining alignment requires separating narrative from structure. A sequence of events can be used as an entry point, but it must be decomposed into variables and relationships that define how the system operates. Each step in the sequence must be translated into a transformation that preserves variable identity and applies defined interactions. This reconstructs the pathway in a way that can be inspected and verified.

A structured model can generate a narrative as a byproduct. It can describe the sequence of events that occur when variables interact under specific conditions. The narrative is then a representation of the underlying structure, not a replacement for it. When the direction is reversed and the narrative becomes the basis for reasoning, the system loses the constraints that define valid transitions.

The narrative fallacy does not produce random error. It produces outputs that feel coherent because they follow a recognizable pattern. This coherence masks the absence of structure. The system appears to understand the process because it can tell a consistent story, but it cannot generate or verify the transitions that would make that story valid.

Overconfidence and Underthinking

A reasoning system produces certainty when the internal model appears stable. It produces accuracy when that model remains aligned with the structure it is meant to represent. These conditions are not equivalent. Overconfidence emerges when the system treats internal stability as evidence of correctness. Underthinking is the mechanism that creates this condition. It reduces the number of variables tracked, compresses relationships, and skips transitions that would normally enforce constraints. The model becomes easier to process, and the reduction in complexity creates the appearance of clarity. That clarity is not derived from preserving structure. It is the result of removing it.

Underthinking begins at the level of representation. Variables are simplified beyond the point where they capture the distinctions required for accurate interaction. A component that should be defined by specific properties is treated as a general category. This reduces the number of elements the system must track, but it also removes the boundaries that differentiate one variable from another. Relationships applied to these simplified variables become generalized. They no longer reflect the conditions under which the interaction actually holds.

The next layer is transition compression. Structured reasoning requires a sequence of transformations that carry variables from premise to conclusion. Underthinking collapses this sequence. Intermediate states are skipped, and relationships are applied in aggregated form. The system moves directly from input to output without maintaining a traceable pathway. This increases speed, but it removes the ability to verify whether each step preserved structure. The conclusion appears coherent because it aligns with the simplified model, not because it follows from a valid sequence of transformations.

Overconfidence arises from the absence of visible conflict within this reduced model. When variables are simplified and relationships are generalized, contradictions are less likely to appear because the system is not tracking the distinctions that would create them. The model becomes internally consistent by construction. The system interprets this consistency as correctness. It does not recognize that the consistency is a result of reduced resolution rather than accurate representation.

Feedback failure reinforces the condition. When the system receives outcomes that appear to confirm its conclusions, it attributes that confirmation to the validity of its process. It does not evaluate whether the pathway that produced the conclusion was structurally sound. If the outcome aligns with expectations, the system increases confidence in the simplified model. If the outcome does not align, the system may adjust the model superficially without reconstructing the missing structure. The underlying process remains unchanged.

In multi-variable systems, underthinking produces systematic error. The interactions between variables depend on conditions that are not represented in the simplified model. The system applies generalized relationships across contexts where they do not hold. Because the model does not track the variables that would reveal the mismatch, the error is not detected at the point of transition. It appears only at the level of outcome, and even then it may be attributed to external factors rather than to the structure of the reasoning process.

Speed amplifies both underthinking and overconfidence. When decisions must be made quickly, the system prioritizes throughput. It reduces the number of variables, compresses relationships, and eliminates validation steps. This produces rapid outputs that appear decisive. The lack of intermediate states removes opportunities for doubt or correction. The system experiences a continuous flow from input to conclusion, which reinforces the perception that the reasoning process is complete.

Overconfidence also alters error handling. When confidence is high, the system is less likely to inspect its own process. It treats conclusions as final rather than as outputs that can be traced and verified. This prevents error localization. When a mismatch occurs, the system may defend the conclusion or adjust peripheral elements rather than examining the transitions that produced it. The absence of inspection allows structural errors to persist and accumulate.

Restoring accuracy requires increasing resolution. Variables must be defined with boundaries that reflect their actual structure, relationships must be applied under the conditions that define them, and transitions must be made explicit. This reintroduces complexity into the model. The system must process more information and maintain more intermediate states. The reduction in speed is a direct consequence of preserving structure.

Confidence then becomes a function of traceability rather than of simplicity. The system can evaluate its conclusions by inspecting the pathway that produced them. If each transition preserves structure and the relationships are applied correctly, confidence is supported by the model. If the pathway contains gaps or inconsistencies, confidence decreases because the system can identify where alignment may have been lost.

False certainty is not the presence of confidence. It is confidence without structural support. It emerges when the system removes the elements that would expose uncertainty and interprets the resulting clarity as accuracy. Eliminating underthinking does not eliminate uncertainty. It makes uncertainty visible by preserving the structure required to detect it.

Chapter 10

Environmental Distortions

A cognitive system does not operate in isolation. It is embedded within an environment that shapes what inputs are available, how frequently they arrive, and how feedback is returned. These environmental conditions do not merely influence behavior at the surface level. They alter the structure of the internal model by changing how variables are formed, how relationships are reinforced, and how transitions are executed. When the environment is aligned with the system's constraints, it supports accurate mapping between internal representation and external conditions. When it is misaligned, it introduces distortions that propagate through every stage of reasoning.

Input structure is the first point of distortion. The system builds its model from the signals it receives. If those signals are incomplete, biased, or unevenly distributed, the variables constructed from them inherit that structure. A variable that should represent a full range of states may instead reflect a narrow subset. Relationships derived from this input will appear consistent within the observed range but will fail when applied outside it. The system does not recognize this limitation because it has no exposure to the missing states.

Frequency and repetition reinforce specific patterns. When certain inputs occur more often than others, the system increases the weight of those patterns within its model. This weighting is not inherently problematic. It becomes a distortion when frequency does not correspond to importance or validity. The system begins to treat repeated patterns as representative of the underlying structure, even if they are artifacts of the environment. This shifts the model toward what is most commonly observed rather than what is most structurally accurate.

Feedback timing further shapes alignment. Immediate feedback allows the system to adjust variables and relationships at the point where they are applied. Delayed feedback separates action from outcome. The system continues to operate based on prior assumptions while the consequences of those actions are still unresolved. When feedback eventually arrives, it must be integrated into a model that has already evolved. This creates layering of error. Corrections are applied to a state that no longer matches the conditions under which the original action was taken.

Noise introduces ambiguity into variable definition. When inputs contain irrelevant or inconsistent signals, the system must determine which components correspond to actual structure and which do not. If noise is not filtered effectively, it becomes incorporated into variables and relationships. The system then models patterns that do not exist in the environment. These patterns may appear stable within the noisy input, but they do not produce accurate predictions when applied to conditions where the noise is absent.

Incentive structures alter evaluation. When outcomes are rewarded based on appearance rather than on process, the system shifts toward producing outputs that satisfy those criteria. This reinforces outcome bias and reduces emphasis on maintaining valid transitions. The system learns to generate conclusions that align with external expectations, even if the pathway that produces them does not preserve structure. Over time, this changes how reasoning is executed at a fundamental level.

Social environments introduce additional layers of distortion. Shared models are often adopted without independent verification. Variables and relationships are inherited from external sources rather than constructed through direct interaction with the environment. If those external models contain errors or simplifications, the system integrates them as if they were accurate representations. This creates alignment within the social group but divergence from the underlying structure those models are meant to describe.

Information density affects processing. High-density environments present more variables and interactions than the system can process with full resolution. To maintain throughput, the system compresses representations, simplifies relationships, and reduces the number of explicit transitions. This allows continued operation under increased load but introduces approximation. The system maintains output production at the cost of structural accuracy.

Over time, these distortions accumulate. The system's internal model drifts from the environment not because the system lacks capability, but because the conditions under which it operates do not support maintaining alignment. Each distortion at the level of input, feedback, or incentive alters how variables and relationships are formed. These alterations compound, producing a model that is internally consistent but externally misaligned.

Correcting environmental distortions requires modifying the conditions under which the system operates. Input must be expanded to include the full range of relevant states. Feedback must be aligned with the timing of actions to allow accurate updates. Noise must be reduced or filtered to prevent incorporation into variables. Incentives must be structured to reinforce valid processes rather than superficial outcomes. Social inputs must be evaluated against external conditions rather than accepted as given.

A system cannot maintain alignment if its environment continuously introduces distortion. Structural accuracy depends on the quality of the signals used to build and update the model. When those signals are controlled, the system can preserve variable definitions, apply relationships correctly, and maintain valid transitions. When they are not, the system adapts to the environment in a way that prioritizes function within that environment over alignment with the underlying structure it is meant to represent.

Information Overload

A cognitive system depends on separating signal from noise before it can construct variables or apply relationships. Signal provides structure. It carries information about how components behave and interact. Noise introduces variation that does not correspond to that structure. When input volume increases beyond the system's processing capacity, this separation degrades. The system does not stop receiving information. It loses the ability to distinguish which parts of that information should be encoded into the model and which should be discarded.

The failure begins at intake. Each input must be evaluated for relevance and mapped to an existing variable or used to define a new one. Under high load, this evaluation is compressed. Inputs are accepted without full filtering, and distinctions between relevant and irrelevant features are reduced. Variables begin to incorporate mixed signals. Their boundaries expand to include elements that do not belong to the same underlying structure. Once this occurs, every interaction that involves those variables carries embedded noise.

As variables degrade, relationships follow. Interactions are defined based on observed patterns between variables. If those variables contain noise, the relationships derived from them reflect both signal and noise simultaneously. The system encodes correlations that do not represent actual interactions. These relationships may appear stable because the noise is consistently present in the input environment, but they fail when applied outside that context. The model becomes tuned to the input stream rather than to the structure it is meant to represent.

Throughput constraints force compression. The system cannot process each input with full resolution when the rate of information exceeds capacity. It reduces detail by collapsing variables, simplifying relationships, and skipping intermediate transitions. This maintains output generation but removes the mechanisms that would normally filter noise. The system continues to produce conclusions, but those conclusions are based on a reduced representation that cannot preserve the distinctions required for accuracy.

Noise accumulation produces drift. Each time a variable incorporates irrelevant elements, the system moves further from the structure it is attempting to model. This drift is incremental. Individual additions of noise may not produce visible errors, but over time the accumulation alters the behavior of the variable. Relationships that were once valid become less precise because they are now applied to a broader, less defined structure. The system adapts to this degraded representation and begins to treat it as normal.

Feedback becomes less effective under these conditions. When outputs are compared to outcomes, the system receives a signal that includes both the effects of valid structure and the effects of noise. It cannot easily separate these components. Corrections are applied to the combined signal, which may reinforce noise rather than eliminate it. This creates a feedback loop where noise is continuously integrated into the model instead of being filtered out.

Attention fragmentation contributes to the breakdown. When inputs arrive from multiple sources with different structures and levels of relevance, the system must switch contexts frequently. Each switch reduces the continuity of processing. Variables defined in one context are partially carried into another, where they may not apply. This blending of contexts introduces additional noise because the system does not fully reset or isolate variables between domains.

As signal-to-noise ratio decreases, confidence does not necessarily decrease with it. The system may continue to produce outputs that appear coherent because the internal model remains consistent with the input stream. The problem is that the input stream itself is not aligned with the underlying structure. The system is accurate relative to its inputs but inaccurate relative to the environment those inputs are meant to represent.

Restoring signal integrity requires reducing input to a level that can be processed with full resolution. Variables must be redefined by isolating the components that correspond to actual structure and removing those that do not. Relationships must be recalibrated based on these refined variables. This process cannot occur while the system is operating at maximum throughput. It requires a reduction in input volume to allow for reconstruction of the model.

Filtering must be reintroduced as an explicit step. Each input is evaluated before integration. Features that do not correspond to defined variables are excluded rather than incorporated. This restores boundary integrity and prevents further accumulation of noise. Over time, the model regains alignment as variables and relationships reflect signal rather than mixed input.

Information overload is not a failure of capacity alone. It is a failure of discrimination under conditions of excess input. The system continues to function, but it functions on a degraded representation where noise is treated as structure. Reducing noise and restoring the ability to distinguish signal allows the system to rebuild variables and relationships that correspond to the environment, reestablishing alignment between input, model, and output.

Social Reinforcement of Error

A cognitive system maintains alignment by comparing its internal model to external conditions. When that comparison is replaced with agreement from other systems operating under the same distortions, error becomes stable. Social reinforcement does not require accuracy. It requires consistency across participants. When multiple systems share similar inputs, constraints, and compression patterns, they converge on the same outputs. This convergence is interpreted as validation, even when the shared model is misaligned with the structure it is meant to represent.

The process begins with model synchronization. Individuals within a group exchange variables and relationships through communication. These elements are adopted without reconstructing the underlying structure. A term is accepted with its implied meaning, and a relationship is accepted with its implied conditions. Because these elements are not independently defined, their boundaries remain ambiguous. The group operates on a shared set of representations that appear stable because they are used consistently across participants.

Repetition reinforces these shared representations. Each time a variable or relationship is expressed and accepted, its perceived validity increases. This reinforcement does not depend on correspondence with external conditions. It depends on frequency within the group. The system begins to weight internally repeated patterns more heavily than externally verified ones. Over time, the group model becomes self-referential. It is validated by its own use rather than by interaction with the environment.

Ambiguity accelerates this process. When variables lack precise boundaries, different participants can interpret them in slightly different ways while still using the same label. This allows agreement to occur at the surface level even when underlying representations differ. The group appears aligned, but the alignment is based on shared language rather than shared structure. Relationships built on these variables inherit the ambiguity, allowing them to be applied across contexts without explicit conditions.

Dissent is filtered through social constraints. A system that produces an output inconsistent with the group model introduces a potential correction signal. For that signal to be integrated, the group must evaluate it against external conditions. If evaluation is based on agreement instead, the signal is rejected or modified to fit the existing model. This prevents the introduction of new variables or relationships that could restore alignment. The group maintains internal consistency by excluding inputs that would require structural change.

Incentive structures reinforce conformity. When acceptance within the group depends on producing outputs that align with the shared model, systems adjust their processing to match those expectations. This shifts evaluation from structural validity to social compatibility. The reasoning chain is compressed or altered to produce conclusions that fit the group's patterns. Over time, this changes how inference is executed. The system prioritizes outputs that will be accepted rather than outputs that preserve structure.

Feedback loops within the group amplify error. Outputs generated by one system become inputs for others. If those outputs contain distortions, the distortions are propagated and reinforced. Each iteration increases the weight of the shared model. Because the group is not referencing external conditions at each step, there is no mechanism to filter out accumulated error. The model becomes more stable internally while diverging further from the environment.

As the group model stabilizes, it becomes resistant to correction. Variables and relationships are treated as fixed because they are consistently reinforced. Introducing a change requires not only modifying the model but also overcoming the inertia of repeated validation. This increases the cost of correction. Systems are less likely to initiate structural updates because those updates conflict with the established model and the incentives that maintain it.

The result is a closed system of validation. Agreement replaces verification. Consistency replaces accuracy. The group maintains a coherent internal model that produces predictable outputs, but those outputs are not constrained by the structure of the environment. The system functions effectively within the group context while failing to map to external conditions.

Restoring alignment requires reintroducing external constraints. Variables must be defined against observable structure rather than against shared language. Relationships must be validated through interaction with the environment, not through repetition within the group. Dissent must be treated as a potential correction signal and evaluated based on its correspondence to external conditions rather than on its alignment with the group model.

Independence at the level of model construction becomes necessary. Each system must be able to reconstruct variables and relationships from primary inputs rather than inheriting them. This does not eliminate communication, but it changes its role. Shared models are compared against independently constructed ones, allowing discrepancies to be identified and resolved based on structure rather than agreement.

Social reinforcement of error does not produce obvious failure in the short term. It produces stable outputs that appear validated through consensus. The divergence becomes visible only when the model is applied to conditions outside the group's shared environment. At that point, the lack of external alignment is exposed because the system has been operating within a closed loop that prioritizes agreement over structure.

Incentives That Reward Wrong Thinking

A system does not optimize for correctness by default. It optimizes for what its feedback loop rewards. Incentives define which outputs are reinforced, which pathways are repeated, and which internal structures are preserved or discarded. When incentives are aligned with structural accuracy, the system strengthens variables, relationships, and transitions that maintain correspondence with reality. When incentives are misaligned, the system strengthens pathways that produce rewarded outputs even if those pathways distort the model. The result is not random error. It is consistent, repeatable misalignment shaped by the reward structure itself.

Incentives operate at the level of evaluation. Every output is implicitly or explicitly judged, and that judgment determines whether the process that produced it is reinforced. If evaluation focuses on appearance, speed, agreement, or short-term outcome, the system adapts to maximize those criteria. It reduces processing steps, compresses variables, and generalizes relationships because these changes increase throughput and improve surface-level coherence. The reasoning chain becomes shorter and less constrained. Outputs are produced efficiently, but the transformations that would normally preserve structure are no longer enforced.

This adaptation is not optional. Once a pathway produces a rewarded outcome, the system increases its likelihood of reuse. Over time, these pathways become dominant. Structured inference, which requires more time and maintains more intermediate states, is used less frequently because it is not consistently rewarded. The system reallocates its resources toward processes that produce outputs aligned with the incentive structure, not toward processes that preserve alignment with the underlying model.

Misaligned incentives also alter variable formation. When certain types of outputs are rewarded, the system begins to define variables in a way that supports those outputs. Boundaries are adjusted to include or exclude components that make the desired conclusion easier to produce. This changes the structure of the model at its foundation. Relationships derived from these variables reflect the modified definitions rather than the actual structure of the environment.

Relationship distortion follows. Interactions are applied in ways that support the rewarded outcome, even if the conditions required for those interactions are not present. The system generalizes relationships because specificity limits the range of outputs that can be produced. By removing conditions, the system increases flexibility. This flexibility allows it to generate conclusions that align with incentives across a wider range of inputs, but it reduces the accuracy of those conclusions.

Feedback loops reinforce the distortion. When outputs that match incentives are consistently rewarded, the system receives a signal that its process is effective. It does not distinguish between outputs produced through valid transitions and those produced through compressed or altered pathways. The reinforcement applies to the entire sequence, strengthening the use of invalid transitions alongside valid ones. Over time, the system cannot easily separate the two because they have been learned together.

Short-term incentives produce long-term degradation. When rewards are tied to immediate outcomes, the system prioritizes processes that generate quick results. This often involves skipping validation steps and reducing the resolution of variables and relationships. The immediate output may align with expectations, but the underlying model accumulates error. As conditions change or complexity increases, the system's performance declines because the structure required to handle those conditions has been degraded.

Social incentives amplify the effect. When acceptance, status, or agreement are tied to producing certain outputs, the system adjusts its reasoning to match group expectations. This introduces an additional layer of constraint that is independent of structural accuracy. The system must satisfy both the internal model and the external incentive structure. When these conflict, the incentive structure dominates because it provides immediate feedback. The system prioritizes outputs that are rewarded over those that are structurally valid.

Detection of misalignment requires separating outcome from process. A rewarded outcome does not indicate that the reasoning pathway is correct. The system must inspect the variables, relationships, and transitions used to produce the output. If those elements do not preserve structure, the pathway must be rejected even if the outcome is favorable. This prevents reinforcement of processes that degrade the model.

Realignment requires modifying the incentive structure itself. Rewards must be tied to the integrity of the reasoning chain rather than to the surface characteristics of the output. This involves evaluating whether variables are clearly defined, whether relationships are applied within their valid conditions, and whether transitions are traceable and consistent. When these criteria are reinforced, the system adapts by strengthening pathways that maintain structure.

Incentives shape behavior by selecting which processes survive. When they are aligned with structural accuracy, the system evolves toward more precise and reliable reasoning. When they are misaligned, the system evolves toward outputs that satisfy external criteria while diverging from the structure it is meant to represent. The difference between correct and incorrect thinking is therefore not only a matter of knowledge or capability. It is a function of the conditions that determine which forms of reasoning are reinforced over time.

Chapter 11

Reproducibility Failure

A system demonstrates validity when it can produce the same output from the same inputs under the same conditions. Reproducibility is not a secondary property. It is the operational test of whether variables are defined correctly, relationships are applied consistently, and transitions preserve structure. When reproducibility fails, it indicates that one or more components of the reasoning process are unstable. The system may still generate outputs that appear correct, but those outputs cannot be relied on because the pathway that produces them does not hold under repeated execution.

The failure begins with variable inconsistency. If the same input is mapped to different variables across instances, the system is not operating on a fixed representation. Small changes in interpretation alter the starting state of the model. These changes propagate through the reasoning chain, producing different outputs even when the external conditions are unchanged. This instability is often masked because the variations occur at the level of definition rather than at the level of observable input.

Relationship variability compounds the issue. Interactions must be applied under defined conditions with consistent parameters. When those conditions are not explicitly maintained, the system may apply the same relationship differently across instances. This can occur through implicit adjustments in scope, timing, or magnitude. The relationship appears stable in description but varies in execution. The system produces outputs that diverge because the transformations applied are not identical, even though they are labeled as such.

Transition inconsistency introduces further divergence. Each step in the reasoning chain must be executed in the same sequence with the same operations. When steps are skipped, reordered, or compressed differently across instances, the pathway from input to output changes. Even if each individual step is valid, altering the sequence changes the state of the variables at each stage. The final output reflects these differences, leading to variation in results.

Hidden variables are a central source of reproducibility failure. These are factors that influence the system but are not explicitly represented in the model. They alter variable states or relationships without being tracked. Because they are not part of the defined structure, the system cannot control or replicate their effects. Outputs vary depending on the presence or state of these hidden variables, even when the visible inputs remain constant.

Environmental conditions contribute to hidden variability. Differences in input quality, timing, or context alter how variables are formed and how relationships are applied. If these conditions are not standardized or accounted for, the system operates under different constraints in each instance. The reasoning process appears the same, but the underlying conditions differ, leading to inconsistent outputs.

Compression increases variability. When the reasoning chain is reduced to fewer explicit steps, the internal operations that produce the output are not fully specified. This allows variation in how those operations are executed. The system fills in the missing steps based on context or prior patterns, which may differ across instances. The output becomes dependent on implicit processes that are not controlled or reproducible.

Outcome-based validation obscures the problem. If outputs are evaluated only by whether they appear correct, variability in the pathway is not detected. The system may produce the correct result in one instance and an incorrect result in another, but without inspecting the process, the difference is attributed to external factors or randomness.

The underlying inconsistency in variables, relationships, or transitions remains unaddressed.

Reproducibility requires explicit control over the entire chain. Variables must be defined in a way that produces the same representation for the same input. Relationships must be applied with fixed conditions and parameters. Transitions must be executed in a consistent sequence with no hidden variation. Environmental conditions must be either controlled or incorporated into the model as explicit variables. This reduces the number of uncontrolled factors that can influence the output.

Verification depends on repetition. The system must execute the same reasoning process multiple times under the same conditions to confirm that the output remains stable. When variation occurs, the system must trace the chain to identify which component changed. This allows for targeted correction, restoring consistency at the point of divergence.

Reproducibility failure is not a minor inconsistency. It indicates that the system's internal structure is not stable enough to support reliable reasoning. Without reproducibility, conclusions cannot be trusted because they are not consistently derived from the same conditions. Restoring reproducibility restores control over the reasoning process, ensuring that outputs reflect the structure of the model rather than variation in how that model is applied.

Inconsistent Reasoning Outputs

A system produces inconsistent outputs when it does not preserve the same internal state and transformation sequence for identical inputs. The input may appear unchanged at the surface level, but the system is not operating on a fixed representation. Differences arise because variables are defined differently across instances, relationships are applied with variation, or transitions are executed through different pathways. The conclusion is not determined solely by the input. It is determined by how the system constructs and processes that input at the moment of reasoning.

The first point of divergence is variable formation. An input must be mapped to defined variables before any transformation can occur. If this mapping is unstable, the system begins from a different initial state each time. A term may be interpreted with slightly different boundaries, including or excluding components depending on context, memory, or recent exposure. These changes are often small, but they alter the structure of the model. Because every subsequent step depends on the initial variable definitions, the final output reflects these early differences.

Relationship application introduces further variability. Interactions between variables must be applied under consistent conditions. When those conditions are not explicitly maintained, the system may adjust how a relationship is used. The same interaction may be treated as strong in one instance and weak in another, or as conditional in one context and unconditional in another. These shifts change how variables influence each other, producing different intermediate states even when the starting variables are similar.

Transition pathways determine how the system moves from premise to conclusion. In a stable system, this pathway is fixed. Each step follows a defined sequence, and the same operations are applied in the same order. When transitions are compressed or partially reconstructed, the system fills in missing steps based on context. This reconstruction is not deterministic. It depends on recent patterns, cognitive load, and environmental cues. As a result, the pathway differs across instances, leading to different conclusions.

Hidden state variables amplify inconsistency. These include factors such as prior exposure, emotional state, attention allocation, and environmental context. They influence how variables are defined and how relationships are applied, but they are not explicitly represented in the model. Because they are not controlled, their effects vary between instances. The system produces different outputs because it is operating under different internal conditions, even though the external input is the same.

Feedback history also alters processing. Previous outcomes influence how the system evaluates current inputs. If a similar input previously produced a particular result, the system may bias its processing toward that result. This introduces path dependence. The current output is influenced not only by the present input but also by the sequence of prior states that led to the current configuration of the model.

Compression increases variability by removing explicit structure. When the system does not maintain intermediate states, it cannot ensure that each transformation is applied consistently. The reasoning chain becomes a set of approximations rather than a defined sequence. Small differences in approximation accumulate, producing divergent outputs. The system appears to be applying the same process, but the underlying operations differ in detail.

Detection of inconsistency requires comparing the full reasoning chain across instances. It is not sufficient to compare inputs and outputs. The system must examine how variables were defined, which relationships were applied, and how transitions were executed. Differences at any of these levels can produce divergence. Identifying the point of variation allows the system to stabilize that component.

Stabilization involves constraining each stage of the process. Variable definitions must be explicit and consistently applied. Relationships must include the conditions under which they operate. Transition sequences must be preserved without omission or reordering. Hidden variables must be either controlled or incorporated into the model so that their influence can be accounted for. This reduces the degrees of freedom within the system, limiting the pathways through which variability can be introduced.

Consistency is not achieved by forcing the same conclusion. It is achieved by ensuring that the same structured process is applied to the same input. When the process is stable, the output becomes stable because it is determined by a fixed chain of transformations. When the process varies, the output varies because the system is effectively solving a different problem each time, even if the input appears unchanged.

Lack of Process Stability

A reasoning system produces stable outputs only when the process that generates those outputs is fixed. Process stability means that identical inputs move through the same sequence of defined transformations, with variables retaining their boundaries, relationships applied under consistent conditions, and transitions executed in a controlled order. When this structure is not maintained, the system does not operate as a single model. It operates as a set of loosely connected pathways that produce different results depending on how they are assembled in each instance.

Instability begins with variation in execution. Even when variables and relationships are defined, the system may not apply them in a consistent sequence. Steps are skipped, reordered, or partially reconstructed based on context. Each variation alters the state of the system at intermediate stages. Because later transformations depend on these states, small differences early in the chain produce larger differences at the conclusion. The output reflects the pathway taken, not just the input provided.

This variation is often introduced through implicit processing. When parts of the reasoning chain are not explicitly represented, the system fills in the missing steps using pattern completion. These implicit steps are not fixed. They depend on recent exposure, cognitive load, and environmental cues. The same input can trigger different internal completions across instances, leading to different transformation sequences. The system appears to be applying the same logic, but the underlying operations differ.

Variable instability contributes to process variation. If variables are not defined with strict boundaries, their representation can shift between instances. The system begins each reasoning sequence from a slightly different state. Relationships applied to these variables produce different effects because the inputs to those relationships are not identical. Even if the sequence of steps is preserved, the outputs diverge because the elements being transformed are not consistent.

Relationship inconsistency further disrupts stability. Interactions must be applied with fixed parameters and conditions. When those conditions are not enforced, the system adjusts how relationships are used based on context. This introduces variability into each transformation. The same step produces different results because the relationship is not executed in the same way each time.

Hidden dependencies amplify instability. Factors such as attention, prior state, and environmental context influence how the system processes information. When these factors are not controlled or represented, they introduce variation into the reasoning process. The system operates under different internal conditions across instances, even when the external input is unchanged. This creates divergence that cannot be accounted for within the defined model.

Compression removes the structure required for repeatability. When the system reduces the number of explicit steps, it also removes the constraints that ensure those steps are applied consistently. The reasoning process becomes a series of approximations rather than a defined sequence. Each approximation introduces degrees of freedom that allow variation. The system can reach similar conclusions through different pathways, but it cannot guarantee that the same pathway will be used each time.

The absence of validation at intermediate steps allows instability to persist. If the system does not verify each transformation, it cannot detect when a step deviates from its defined operation. Errors introduced at one stage are carried forward without correction. Because the pathway is not inspected, the system has no mechanism to enforce consistency across instances.

Stability requires explicit control over the process. Each stage must be defined and executed in a way that can be repeated without variation. Variables must be constructed identically from the same input. Relationships must be applied with the same conditions and parameters. Transitions must follow a fixed sequence, with no implicit steps or reordering. Environmental and internal factors that influence processing must be either stabilized or incorporated into the model.

Repeatability emerges from constraint. By limiting the ways in which the system can process an input, the number of possible pathways is reduced. The system is forced to use the same sequence of operations each time. This does not reduce capability. It ensures that the capability is applied consistently.

Without process stability, outputs cannot be trusted as representations of the model. They are products of variable execution rather than of defined structure. Restoring stability restores the connection between input, process, and output, allowing the system to produce results that are not only accurate but also reproducible across instances.

The Inability to Improve

A system improves only when it can detect where it failed, isolate the component responsible, and update that component without disrupting the rest of the structure. When any part of this sequence breaks, error does not resolve. It stabilizes. The system continues to produce outputs, but the internal model does not change in a way that reduces future error. What appears as repeated mistakes is not a failure of effort. It is a failure of the architecture required for correction.

The first barrier is detection. A system must recognize that an output does not align with external conditions. If evaluation is based on internal coherence, group agreement, or short-term outcomes, incorrect outputs can appear acceptable. Without a reliable signal that distinguishes correct from incorrect, the system has no trigger to initiate correction. Error becomes invisible because the criteria used to evaluate it do not reflect the structure of the environment.

Even when a mismatch is detected, localization is often absent. The system observes that the output is incorrect but cannot identify which part of the reasoning chain produced the deviation. Variables may be ambiguous, relationships loosely defined, and transitions compressed. Without a clear pathway from input to output, the system cannot trace where structure was altered. Correction becomes diffuse. Multiple components are adjusted without isolating the source, and the underlying error remains embedded in the model.

Feedback timing further limits improvement. When consequences are delayed, the system cannot associate the outcome with the specific process that produced it. By the time feedback is received, the internal state has changed. The system attempts to update a model that no longer matches the conditions under which the error occurred. This weakens the connection between action and correction, reducing the effectiveness of feedback as a mechanism for improvement.

Incentive structures can reinforce persistence of error. If outputs that align with external expectations are rewarded regardless of the process used, the system strengthens the pathways that produce those outputs. Even when those pathways contain invalid transitions, they are repeated because they achieve the rewarded result. The system optimizes for the incentive, not for structural accuracy. Error persists because it is embedded within the pathways that are being reinforced.

Compression prevents structural refinement. Improvement requires inspecting and adjusting individual components of the reasoning chain. When the process is compressed, these components are not explicitly represented. The system cannot modify what it cannot see. It may attempt to adjust the overall output, but without access to intermediate states, it cannot refine the variables, relationships, or transitions that produced it. The model remains unchanged at the level where correction is needed.

Hidden variables introduce uncontrolled variation. Factors that influence the system but are not represented in the model alter how inputs are processed and how relationships are applied. When an error occurs, the system cannot determine whether it resulted from the defined structure or from these hidden influences. This uncertainty prevents targeted correction. The system may adjust visible components while the hidden source of variation remains.

Reinforcement of prior patterns stabilizes error over time. Each time a pathway is used, its likelihood of reuse increases. If that pathway contains a structural flaw, the flaw is repeated and strengthened. The system becomes more efficient at producing the same incorrect transformation. This creates a form of stability where the error is consistently reproduced. The system appears reliable, but it is reliably misaligned.

Lack of variable clarity prevents refinement. When variables are not defined with precise boundaries, adjustments to those variables are ambiguous. The system cannot determine how a change in definition will affect relationships or outcomes. This discourages modification. The system maintains existing definitions because altering them would introduce uncertainty across the model. Error persists because the structure that produces it is not being redefined.

Improvement requires restoring the full correction loop. Detection must be based on alignment with external conditions rather than on internal coherence. Localization must identify the first invalid transition in the reasoning chain. Correction must adjust the specific variable, relationship, or transition at that point and propagate the change forward. Feedback must be timed and structured to connect outcomes with the processes that produced them. Incentives must reinforce pathways that preserve structure rather than those that produce acceptable outputs through compression or distortion.

When this loop is intact, the system reduces error over time because each mismatch leads to a targeted update. When the loop is broken, error becomes part of the system's stable behavior. The system continues to operate, but it does not converge toward accuracy. It cycles through the same transformations, producing variations of the same misalignment without altering the structure that generates them.

PART IV

BUILDING THE LOGIC ENGINE

Chapter 12

Reintroducing Structure

A system regains alignment when it restores the conditions that allow variables, relationships, and transitions to remain stable across time. This is not a matter of adding new information. It is a matter of reorganizing how existing information is represented and processed so that structure is preserved from input to output. Reintroducing structure means constraining the system so that each step in the reasoning chain operates on defined elements under known conditions, with no hidden variation or implicit transformation.

The process begins with reconstruction of variables. Each variable must correspond to a specific component with boundaries that do not shift during processing. This requires removing compressed or overloaded terms that contain multiple structures and separating them into distinct elements. The system must be able to identify what is included within each variable and what is excluded. Without this separation, interactions cannot be defined with precision because the system does not know which component is being affected at each step.

Once variables are stabilized, relationships must be redefined. Interactions between variables are not general associations. They are conditional transformations that depend on the state of the variables and the context in which they occur. Reintroducing structure requires specifying these conditions explicitly. The system must define when a relationship applies, how it changes the variables involved, and what constraints limit that change. This replaces generalized patterns with defined mechanisms that can be applied consistently.

Transition sequences must then be made explicit. The system must move from premise to conclusion through a series of steps that can be traced and verified. Each transition should represent a single transformation that preserves the identity of the variables and applies a defined relationship. Skipped or implicit steps must be reconstructed so that the full pathway is visible. This allows the system to maintain continuity and to detect where deviations occur.

Constraint enforcement is central to this reconstruction. At each stage, the system must ensure that variables remain within their defined boundaries and that relationships are applied only under valid conditions. This requires active validation. Each transformation is checked against the model before proceeding. If a mismatch is detected, the system halts and corrects the step rather than allowing the error to propagate. This prevents accumulation of distortion across the chain.

Feedback must be integrated into the process at the level of structure rather than at the level of outcome. When a mismatch occurs between the system's output and external conditions, the system must trace the reasoning chain to identify the first point of divergence. Correction is applied at that point, and the sequence is recalculated from there. This ensures that the update modifies the structure that produced the error rather than adjusting the output without addressing its cause.

Environmental conditions must also be aligned with structural processing. Input volume must be reduced to a level that allows full resolution of variables and relationships. Noise must be filtered before integration into the model. Incentives must be adjusted so that they reinforce the use of structured pathways rather than compressed or approximate ones. Without these changes, the system will revert to patterns that degrade structure because those patterns are easier to execute under high load or misaligned incentives.

Reintroducing structure increases processing demand. The system must track more variables, maintain more intermediate states, and apply relationships with greater precision. This reduces throughput in the short term. The tradeoff is that each output is derived from a pathway that preserves alignment with the model. Over time, this produces greater efficiency because the system does not need to correct accumulated error or operate on distorted representations.

Stability emerges as the system consistently applies the same structured process. Variables are constructed in the same way for the same inputs, relationships are applied with fixed conditions, and transitions follow a defined sequence. This repeatability allows the system to produce consistent outputs and to refine its model through targeted correction. Each update improves the structure without introducing additional variability.

Reintroducing structure is not a one-time adjustment. It is a sustained mode of operation. The system must continuously maintain variable clarity, enforce constraints, and validate transitions. When these elements are preserved, reasoning remains anchored to the structure of the environment. Outputs reflect the defined interactions within the model, and the system retains the ability to detect and correct deviations as they occur.

Structured Thinking as System Architecture

A reasoning system functions when its architecture enforces how information is represented, transformed, and verified. Structured thinking is not a technique applied at the surface level. It is the configuration of the system itself. Variables are defined with fixed boundaries, relationships are specified with conditions, and transitions are executed in a sequence that preserves continuity. When this architecture is present, the system produces outputs that are constrained by its structure. When it is absent, outputs are generated through approximation, association, or compression, and the connection between input and conclusion is no longer controlled.

Rebuilding reasoning begins by establishing a stable representation layer. Inputs must be decomposed into variables that correspond to distinct components. Each variable must maintain identity across the reasoning process. This requires eliminating ambiguous terms and replacing them with elements that have defined inclusion and exclusion criteria. The system must be able to track each variable as it moves through transformations without reinterpretation. This layer forms the foundation on which all subsequent operations depend.

The next layer defines interactions. Relationships between variables must specify how changes propagate through the system. This includes direction, magnitude, timing, and conditions under which the interaction applies. These relationships are not inferred during processing. They are part of the architecture. When the system applies them, it does so under the constraints that define them. This ensures that each transformation reflects the behavior encoded in the model rather than an approximation derived from pattern matching.

Execution occurs through a controlled sequence of transitions. Each transition applies a single relationship to a defined set of variables, producing a new state that can be traced to the previous one. The sequence must be explicit. Skipping steps or compressing multiple transformations into one removes the ability to verify whether structure has been preserved. By maintaining discrete transitions, the system ensures that each change in state is accounted for and can be inspected if a mismatch occurs.

Constraint enforcement operates across all layers. Variables must remain within their defined boundaries, relationships must be applied only under valid conditions, and transitions must follow the sequence that maintains continuity. This enforcement is active. The system checks each step before proceeding. If a variable shifts or a relationship is misapplied, the process is corrected at that point. This prevents the propagation of error and maintains alignment between the internal model and the structure it represents.

Feedback integration connects the architecture to external conditions. Outputs are compared to observed results, and discrepancies trigger a trace through the reasoning chain. The system identifies the first transition where the transformation deviated from the model and adjusts that component. This targeted correction updates the architecture without altering unrelated elements. Over time, this process refines the model, increasing its accuracy and stability.

Scalability emerges from hierarchical organization. As the number of variables and interactions increases, the system groups them into subsystems. Each subsystem maintains its own structure while interacting with others through defined interfaces. This allows the system to manage complexity without losing clarity. Lower-level interactions define local behavior, while higher-level interactions coordinate the system as a whole. The architecture remains consistent across levels, preserving the same principles of variable definition, relationship specification, and transition control.

Rebuilding reasoning also requires controlling environmental inputs. High input volume, noise, and misaligned incentives push the system toward compression and approximation. To maintain structure, the system must operate under conditions that allow full resolution of variables and relationships. This includes filtering inputs, aligning feedback with the timing of actions, and reinforcing processes that preserve structure rather than those that maximize speed or agreement.

The result of this reconstruction is not a change in what the system knows. It is a change in how the system uses what it knows. Information is no longer processed as loosely connected elements. It is organized into a framework where each component has a defined role and interacts with others under specified conditions. Outputs are produced through a pathway that can be traced, verified, and corrected.

Structured thinking restores control. The system no longer relies on patterns that happen to produce acceptable results. It operates on an architecture that constrains how conclusions are formed. This allows it to maintain alignment across different conditions, to handle increased complexity without collapse, and to improve through targeted correction. Reasoning becomes a function of the system's structure rather than a byproduct of its inputs or its prior patterns.

Standardizing the Thought Process

A system produces repeatable outputs when the process that generates those outputs is fixed at the level of structure. Standardization does not mean simplifying thought into rigid templates. It means defining how variables are constructed, how relationships are applied, and how transitions are executed so that the same input moves through the same sequence of operations every time. The goal is not uniform conclusions across all contexts. The goal is uniform processing, where differences in output arise from differences in input, not from variation in execution.

The first requirement is consistent input construction. Raw information must be translated into variables using the same criteria on every pass. This includes defining boundaries, separating composite terms into discrete elements, and assigning each variable a stable representation. If input construction varies, the system begins each reasoning sequence from a different state. Even with identical external inputs, the internal model is altered before processing begins, which makes repeatability impossible. Standardization starts at the point where information enters the system.

Once variables are constructed, relationships must be applied using fixed rules. Each interaction should have defined conditions and a consistent method of transformation. The system cannot adjust how a relationship operates based on context unless that adjustment is itself part of the defined conditions. This removes interpretive flexibility at the level of execution. The relationship either applies under its conditions or it does not. When it applies, it produces the same transformation given the same inputs. This creates stability across instances.

Transition sequencing must also be standardized. The order in which relationships are applied determines the intermediate states of the system. Changing the sequence changes those states, which changes the final output. A repeatable model enforces a fixed pathway from premise to conclusion. Each step is executed in the same position within the sequence, and each step produces a defined state that feeds into the next. This eliminates variation caused by reordering or skipping transformations.

Intermediate state tracking preserves continuity. After each transition, the system must maintain a record of the current state of all variables. This allows the process to be inspected and ensures that subsequent transformations operate on the correct inputs. Without this tracking, the system relies on reconstruction or approximation of prior states, which introduces variation. Standardization requires that each state be explicitly maintained and passed forward through the sequence.

Validation at each stage enforces consistency. After applying a relationship, the system checks whether the resulting state conforms to the defined structure. Variables must remain within their boundaries, and the transformation must match the conditions of the relationship. If a deviation occurs, it is corrected before the process continues. This prevents divergence from accumulating across steps and ensures that each stage of the model remains aligned with its definitions.

Context control reduces hidden variation. External factors such as cognitive load, environmental noise, and prior state influence how the system processes information. Standardization requires minimizing these influences or incorporating them into the model. If they remain unaccounted for, they introduce variability into input construction, relationship application, and transition sequencing. A repeatable model operates under conditions that allow the defined process to be executed without interference.

Compression must be limited to preserve structure. When multiple steps are collapsed into a single transformation, the system loses visibility into how the output was produced. This prevents verification and introduces variation because the compressed step can be executed differently across instances. Standardization maintains explicit transitions, even when the system becomes efficient at executing them. Efficiency is achieved through familiarity with the sequence, not through removal of structure.

Feedback integration completes the model. Outputs are compared to external conditions, and discrepancies trigger a trace through the standardized process. Because each step is fixed, the system can identify exactly where the transformation diverged. Correction is applied at that point, and the model is updated in a way that preserves the rest of the structure. Over time, this produces convergence, where repeated execution of the same process yields increasingly accurate outputs.

A repeatable model does not eliminate flexibility. It defines where flexibility exists. Variation is allowed in the input, and the model adapts through feedback-driven updates to its structure. What remains fixed is the way the system processes information. This separation allows the system to handle new conditions without losing stability. The process remains constant while the model evolves.

Standardizing the thought process transforms reasoning from an adaptive but inconsistent activity into a controlled system. Each output can be traced to a defined pathway, each deviation can be localized and corrected, and each update improves the structure without introducing new variability. The system becomes reliable not because it produces the same answers, but because it produces answers through the same architecture every time.

Traceable Reasoning

A reasoning system becomes controllable when each transformation from input to output is exposed and preserved. Traceability requires that every variable, relationship, and transition be represented in a way that can be inspected after execution. The system must be able to show how an input was decomposed, how each component interacted with others, and how those interactions produced the final state. Without this visibility, outputs exist without a pathway, and there is no mechanism to determine whether they were produced through valid structure or through approximation.

The process begins with explicit variable construction. Inputs are not carried forward as raw or composite forms. They are decomposed into elements with defined boundaries, and each element is assigned a stable representation. This allows the system to track how each component changes across the reasoning sequence. If a variable is altered, the system records both its prior state and the transformation applied. This creates a chain of states that can be followed step by step.

Relationships must be applied in a way that is both defined and observable. Each interaction between variables is executed under specified conditions, and the effect of that interaction is recorded. The system must capture not only that a relationship was applied, but why it was applied and how it altered the variables involved. This includes the conditions that triggered the relationship and the resulting change in state. By doing this, the system ensures that each transformation is tied to a defined rule rather than to implicit pattern matching.

Transitions form the backbone of traceability. Each step in the reasoning sequence represents a discrete change from one state to another. These steps must be preserved in order, with no compression or omission. The system maintains a sequence where each transition is linked to the previous one, forming a continuous chain from premise to conclusion. If a transition is skipped or combined with others, the chain is broken, and the system loses the ability to reconstruct how the output was generated.

Intermediate state preservation is necessary for full visibility. After each transition, the system records the current configuration of all variables. This allows the entire reasoning pathway to be replayed or inspected at any point. If an error is detected in the final output, the system can move backward through these states to identify where the divergence occurred. Without these records, the system must infer prior states, which introduces uncertainty and prevents precise localization of error.

Constraint tracking ensures that each step adheres to the model. As variables are transformed, the system verifies that they remain within their defined boundaries and that relationships are applied under valid conditions. These checks are part of the trace. They show not only the transformations that occurred but also that those transformations were valid according to the model. If a constraint is violated, the trace captures that violation, allowing the system to identify and correct the specific step responsible.

Traceability also exposes hidden variation. Factors that influence processing but are not explicitly represented in the model become visible when their effects appear as unexplained changes in the trace. If the same input produces different sequences or states across instances, the trace reveals where the pathways diverge. This allows the system to identify and incorporate previously hidden variables or to stabilize conditions that are introducing variation.

The structure of the trace must be consistent. Each reasoning sequence should produce a pathway that follows the same format, with variables constructed in the same way, relationships applied in the same order, and transitions recorded using the same representation. This consistency allows traces from different instances to be compared directly. Differences in output can then be linked to differences in input or to specific changes in the reasoning chain, rather than to variation in how the trace itself is constructed.

Traceable reasoning transforms outputs into inspectable artifacts. Each conclusion is accompanied by a pathway that shows how it was produced. This allows verification, where the system checks that each step follows from the previous one under the defined relationships. It allows correction, where errors are localized and adjusted at the point of divergence. It also allows learning, where repeated traces reveal patterns of failure or success that can be used to refine the model.

Making thinking visible does not slow the system in a way that reduces capability. It replaces unobserved variation with controlled execution. The system may process fewer inputs in a given time, but each output is derived from a pathway that can be trusted, inspected, and improved. Over time, this increases efficiency because the system no longer spends resources correcting accumulated errors or reconciling inconsistent outputs.

A reasoning system that cannot expose its own process cannot maintain alignment. Traceability restores the link between structure and output by ensuring that every transformation is recorded and verifiable. The system becomes capable of maintaining consistency, identifying deviation, and refining its architecture through direct observation of how it operates.

Chapter 13

Model Construction

A model is a constructed representation of how variables interact under defined conditions to produce outcomes. It is not a collection of facts or observations. It is an organized structure that maps components, specifies their relationships, and constrains how changes propagate through the system. Model construction begins when the system stops treating information as isolated inputs and starts organizing it into a framework that can generate predictions through controlled transformation.

The foundation of a model is variable definition. Each variable represents a component that can change state. For the model to function, these variables must be bounded, meaning their identity does not shift during processing. This requires separating composite ideas into discrete elements and removing ambiguity from their definitions. A variable must correspond to something that can be tracked across transformations. If its meaning changes mid-process, the model loses continuity, and relationships applied to it no longer produce reliable effects.

Once variables are defined, the model must establish relationships. These relationships describe how one variable influences another under specific conditions. They are directional and conditional. A relationship may apply only when a variable is within a certain range or when another variable is in a particular state. Model construction requires specifying these conditions so that the relationship is not applied arbitrarily. Each interaction must be predictable given the state of the system.

State representation is the next layer. At any point in the reasoning process, the system must be able to describe the current configuration of all variables. This state is the result of prior transformations and serves as the input for the next step. Without explicit state representation, the model cannot maintain continuity. It cannot determine how past changes influence current behavior, and it cannot project forward in a controlled way.

Transition rules define how the model moves from one state to another. Each transition applies one or more relationships to the current state, producing a new state. These transitions must be structured so that they preserve the identity of variables and the conditions of relationships. The model must specify the order in which transitions occur, because different sequences produce different outcomes. By defining this order, the model ensures that its behavior is consistent across instances.

Constraint integration limits the range of possible states and transitions. Constraints define what configurations are valid within the model. They prevent variables from entering states that violate the structure of the system and restrict relationships to conditions where they are applicable. Constraints reduce the number of possible pathways, forcing the model to operate within a defined space. This is what allows the model to produce reliable outputs rather than a wide range of inconsistent results.

Model construction also requires handling incomplete information. Real inputs are rarely fully specified. The model must define how to operate when variables are partially known. This may involve assigning provisional states, maintaining ranges, or deferring certain transitions until more information is available. The key is that these approaches are defined within the model. The system does not fill gaps through uncontrolled inference. It uses structured methods that preserve consistency.

Validation connects the model to external conditions. After the model produces an output, that output is compared to observed outcomes. If there is a mismatch, the model must identify which variable, relationship, or transition failed to represent reality accurately. Correction is applied at that point, and the model is updated. This process refines the structure over time, increasing its ability to produce outputs that align with the environment.

Scalability requires hierarchical organization. As the number of variables and relationships increases, the model groups them into subsystems. Each subsystem maintains its own structure while interacting with others through defined interfaces. This allows the model to handle complexity without losing clarity. Lower-level models describe local interactions, while higher-level models coordinate these interactions to produce system-wide behavior.

A constructed model is not static. It evolves as new information is integrated and as corrections are applied. What remains constant is the architecture. Variables remain bounded, relationships remain conditional, transitions remain ordered, and constraints remain enforced. This consistency allows the model to adapt without losing stability.

Model construction transforms reasoning from reactive processing into structured generation. The system no longer responds to inputs by assembling patterns. It produces outputs by applying a defined set of operations to a structured representation of the problem. This allows it to maintain alignment across conditions, to detect and correct error, and to extend its capability without introducing instability.

Building Internal Models of Reality

An internal model is a constructed mapping between the structure of the environment and the structure of the system that represents it. It does not store reality. It encodes how components relate, how changes propagate, and what constraints limit those changes. Building this model requires translating external conditions into variables, defining how those variables interact, and maintaining a state representation that evolves as new inputs are integrated. The goal is not completeness. It is functional alignment, where the model can produce outputs that match how the external system behaves under comparable conditions.

The process begins with segmentation of the environment into components that can be represented as variables. This segmentation is not arbitrary. It must reflect boundaries that exist in the system being modeled. If boundaries are drawn incorrectly, interactions will be misrepresented because the model will apply relationships to elements that do not behave as a unit. Each variable must correspond to a component that maintains identity across changes, allowing the system to track how it evolves over time.

Once variables are established, the model defines interactions. These interactions must capture direction, magnitude, and conditional application. A variable does not influence all others in the same way or under all conditions. The model specifies when an interaction occurs, what triggers it, and how it alters the state of the variables involved. This creates a network where changes in one part of the system propagate through defined pathways rather than through generalized association.

State mapping maintains the current configuration of the system. At any point, the model must represent the values or conditions of all variables. This state is the basis for prediction. When an input alters one or more variables, the model applies its defined interactions to generate a new state. The accuracy of this process depends on how well the current state reflects the actual system. If the state is misrepresented, subsequent transformations will diverge from reality even if the relationships are correctly defined.

Temporal structure is required to map how systems evolve. Changes do not occur simultaneously across all variables. Some interactions are immediate, while others are delayed. The model must represent this timing, allowing it to simulate how the system moves from one state to another over time. Without this, the model collapses dynamic behavior into static relationships, which produces outputs that do not match the sequence of events in the external system.

Constraint mapping limits the range of possible states and transitions. Real systems do not allow all combinations of variable states. Physical, logical, or contextual constraints restrict what configurations can occur. The model must incorporate these limits so that it does not generate states that are invalid. Constraints also define boundaries where behavior changes, such as thresholds where an interaction activates or deactivates.

Abstraction is used to manage complexity, but it must preserve structure. The model cannot represent every detail of the external system, so it groups variables and interactions into higher-level constructs. These abstractions must maintain the relationships that drive system behavior. If abstraction removes critical interactions or merges components that behave differently, the model loses accuracy. Effective abstraction reduces detail while preserving the pathways through which changes propagate.

Feedback integration aligns the model with the environment. Predictions generated by the model are compared to observed outcomes. When discrepancies occur, the model identifies which part of its structure failed to represent the system accurately. This may involve adjusting variable definitions, refining relationships, or updating constraints. The correction is applied at the point of divergence, and the model is recalculated from that point forward. Over time, this process improves alignment between the model and reality.

Internal consistency is necessary but not sufficient. A model can operate without contradiction and still fail to match external behavior. Alignment requires that the structure of the model corresponds to the structure of the system it represents. This is achieved through continuous validation and correction, ensuring that the pathways within the model produce outcomes that match those observed in the environment.

Building internal models transforms reasoning into simulation. Instead of reacting to inputs with isolated responses, the system uses its model to project how changes will propagate through the structure. This allows it to anticipate outcomes, evaluate alternatives, and adjust behavior before external consequences occur. The quality of this capability depends on the accuracy of the mapping, the stability of the variables, and the precision of the relationships that connect them.

A system that maintains an internal model operates with continuity. Each new input updates the existing state rather than replacing it. The model evolves as a coherent structure, allowing past information to inform future behavior. This continuity enables the system to handle complex, multi-variable environments without losing alignment, because each decision is made within the context of a structured representation that reflects how the system behaves.

Variable Identification

A system can only produce accurate outputs if it selects the correct variables to represent the problem. Variable identification determines what enters the model and what is excluded. This step defines the boundaries of the system's representation before any relationships are applied. If the wrong variables are selected, or if relevant variables are omitted, the model operates on an incomplete or distorted structure. The resulting outputs may appear coherent, but they reflect the limitations of the representation rather than the behavior of the underlying system.

Identification begins with separating components that change independently. A variable must correspond to something that can vary without requiring all other elements to change with it. This independence allows the system to track how specific components influence outcomes. When multiple components are combined into a single variable, their individual effects become inseparable. The model loses resolution because it cannot determine which part of the composite variable is responsible for a change in state.

Relevance is determined by influence on the system's behavior. A variable is included when changes in its state alter the outcome through defined relationships. This requires observing how variations propagate through the system. Variables that do not affect the output under the conditions being modeled can be excluded without loss of accuracy. Including them increases complexity without improving the model's ability to generate correct results. The goal is not to capture every detail, but to capture the components that drive change.

Boundary definition stabilizes each variable. Once identified, the variable must have a fixed meaning that does not shift during processing. This includes specifying what is included within the variable and what is not. If boundaries are unclear, the system may reinterpret the variable across different stages of reasoning. This introduces inconsistency because relationships are applied to elements that are not the same from one step to the next. Stable boundaries ensure that each transformation operates on a consistent entity.

Granularity determines the level of detail at which variables are defined. Variables that are too coarse combine distinct components and obscure their interactions. Variables that are too fine increase complexity without providing additional explanatory power. The system must select a level of granularity that preserves the relationships necessary to model behavior while keeping the number of variables manageable. This balance allows the model to remain both accurate and tractable.

Hidden variables introduce uncontrolled variation. These are components that influence the system but are not represented in the model. Their effects appear as unexplained changes in output or as inconsistencies across instances. Identifying these variables requires tracing where the model's predictions diverge from observed outcomes and determining which unrepresented factors could account for the difference. Incorporating these variables into the model reduces uncertainty and improves alignment.

Variable interaction must also be considered during identification. Some variables only influence the system in combination with others. These interactions may not be visible when variables are considered in isolation. The system must detect where combined states produce effects that individual variables do not. This ensures that the model captures not only direct influences but also the conditions under which those influences emerge.

Context defines which variables are relevant at a given time. A variable that is critical in one scenario may have no effect in another. The model must include mechanisms for activating or deactivating variables based on conditions. This prevents the system from applying relationships where they do not belong and reduces unnecessary complexity. Variable identification is therefore dynamic, but the criteria for inclusion and exclusion remain defined.

Measurement and representation determine how variables are encoded. A variable must be represented in a form that allows relationships to be applied consistently. This may involve assigning ranges, states, or categories that reflect how the component behaves. If representation is inconsistent, the same variable may be interpreted differently across instances, which disrupts the application of relationships and reduces repeatability.

Variable identification shapes the entire reasoning process. It defines what the system can see and what it cannot. Every relationship, transition, and output depends on this initial selection. When variables are correctly identified and defined, the model operates on a structure that reflects the system being analyzed. When they are not, the model produces outputs that are internally consistent but externally misaligned, because it is processing an incomplete or distorted representation of reality.

Relationship Mapping

A model becomes functional when it defines how variables influence one another under specific conditions. Relationship mapping establishes the pathways through which changes propagate. It replaces loose association with controlled transformation. Each relationship specifies direction, conditions, and the form of change that occurs when it is applied. Without this structure, variables exist as isolated elements, and the system cannot generate outcomes that reflect how the underlying components interact.

A relationship begins with direction. One variable alters the state of another, or multiple variables combine to produce an effect on a target. Direction must be explicit because reversing it changes the pathway entirely. When direction is unclear, the system may treat correlated variables as interchangeable, applying transformations in the wrong orientation. This produces outputs that appear plausible but do not reflect the actual sequence of influence within the system.

Conditions determine when a relationship applies. A variable does not influence another across all states. Thresholds, ranges, and contextual factors define the boundaries within which the interaction occurs. Mapping these conditions prevents the system from applying relationships in situations where they do not operate. It also allows the model to represent changes in behavior when variables move across these boundaries. The same pair of variables may interact differently depending on their states, and this must be encoded within the relationship.

The form of change specifies how the target variable is altered. This includes magnitude, rate, and whether the effect is additive, multiplicative, or conditional. The system must define what happens to the target variable when the relationship is applied. Without this specification, the transformation becomes approximate, and the system fills in the effect using pattern completion. This introduces variation and reduces repeatability because the same relationship can produce different outcomes across instances.

Relationships are rarely isolated. They form chains where the output of one interaction becomes the input for another. These chains create pathways through which changes move across the system. Mapping these pathways requires preserving the order of interactions, because altering the sequence changes intermediate states and therefore the final outcome. The system must maintain a structured sequence where each relationship is applied in a defined position relative to others.

Interdependence adds complexity to these chains. Variables may influence each other in loops, where the state of one variable affects another, which in turn feeds back into the original. These feedback structures must be mapped explicitly. The system must define how the loop operates, whether it stabilizes, amplifies, or oscillates the variables involved. Without this, the model cannot represent dynamic behavior, and outputs will diverge when feedback effects are present.

Nonlinear interactions must also be encoded. The effect of a relationship may not scale proportionally with changes in the input variable. Small changes may produce minimal effects within one range and large effects within another. Mapping these nonlinearities requires defining how the relationship behaves across different states. This prevents the system from applying a uniform transformation where the actual system behaves differently under varying conditions.

Intersections between relationships create higher-order effects. When multiple relationships act on a variable simultaneously, their combined effect may differ from the sum of their individual contributions. The model must account for these interactions, specifying how concurrent influences are integrated. This ensures that the system does not treat each relationship in isolation when the actual behavior depends on their combined state.

Temporal ordering influences how relationships unfold. Some interactions occur immediately, while others introduce delays. Mapping this timing allows the model to represent sequences where the effect of one relationship becomes visible only after several transitions. Without temporal structure, the model collapses these dynamics into a single step, which removes the ability to track how changes accumulate over time.

Constraint enforcement maintains validity within the chain. Each relationship must be applied only when its conditions are met, and each resulting state must remain within the defined boundaries of the variables. The system must verify these conditions at each step. If a relationship is applied outside its valid range, the resulting state may propagate error through the entire chain. By enforcing constraints, the model preserves alignment at each stage of the process.

Relationship mapping converts a set of variables into a working system. It defines how changes move, where they stop, and how they combine. When these pathways are structured, the system can generate outputs that reflect the behavior of the underlying components. When they are not, the system relies on approximation, producing results that may align in isolated cases but fail when conditions change.

Chapter 14

Feedback Integration

A model remains aligned only when it continuously compares its internal outputs to external conditions and updates its structure based on the differences. Feedback integration is the mechanism that connects the model to reality. It ensures that the system does not operate in isolation, reinforcing internal coherence while drifting away from the environment it is meant to represent. Without feedback, the model stabilizes around its own structure. With feedback, it remains responsive to the behavior of the system it is modeling.

The process begins with measurement of outcomes. After the model generates a prediction or decision, the system observes the resulting state in the environment. This observation must be translated into the same variable structure used within the model. If the external outcome is represented differently from the internal state, the comparison cannot be performed accurately. Consistent representation allows the system to identify where the model's output diverges from what actually occurred.

Error detection occurs when the internal prediction does not match the observed outcome. This mismatch is not treated as a general failure. It is a signal that a specific part of the model does not reflect the system correctly. The system must quantify this difference in terms of its variables and relationships. This transforms the mismatch into a form that can be traced back through the reasoning chain.

Localization identifies where the divergence first appeared. The system traces the sequence of transitions from the initial input to the final output, comparing the expected state at each step to what would have produced the observed outcome. The first point at which these states differ marks the location of the error. This step is critical because it isolates the component that requires adjustment. Without localization, correction becomes diffuse and affects parts of the model that are not responsible for the mismatch.

Correction modifies the structure at the point of divergence. This may involve redefining a variable boundary, adjusting the conditions under which a relationship applies, or altering the form of the transformation. The change must be precise. It must address the identified error without introducing additional variability into other parts of the model. After the modification, the system recalculates the sequence from that point forward to ensure that the update produces outputs that align more closely with observed conditions.

Temporal alignment determines the effectiveness of feedback. When the time between action and outcome is short, the system can associate the result with the specific process that produced it. As delays increase, this association weakens. The system receives feedback after its internal state has changed, making it more difficult to connect the outcome to the original sequence of transitions. Effective feedback integration requires mechanisms to preserve the state of the model at the time of action so that delayed outcomes can still be linked to the correct pathway.

Signal clarity influences how accurately feedback can be applied. External environments often produce noisy data, where multiple factors affect the observed outcome. The system must isolate the portion of the signal that corresponds to the variables and relationships within the model. If noise is treated as signal, the system will adjust its structure based on irrelevant variation. This introduces instability and reduces alignment. Filtering and contextual analysis are required to ensure that only relevant information is used for correction.

Feedback must operate at the level of structure rather than at the level of output. Adjusting outputs without modifying the underlying variables or relationships does not improve the model. It creates a temporary alignment that fails when conditions change. Structural correction ensures that the model produces accurate outputs across different inputs because the pathways that generate those outputs have been refined.

Reinforcement determines which pathways are strengthened. When a sequence of transformations produces an output that aligns with observed conditions, that pathway is reinforced. The system increases its likelihood of using the same sequence in similar situations. This reinforcement must be tied to structural accuracy rather than to superficial success. If the system reinforces pathways that achieve acceptable results through approximation, it will stabilize around processes that are not reliable under varying conditions.

Feedback integration also requires managing conflicting signals. Different observations may suggest different adjustments to the model. The system must evaluate these signals based on their relevance, consistency, and the conditions under which they were observed. Updates are applied in a way that maintains overall coherence while improving alignment. This may involve weighting certain signals more heavily or delaying updates until sufficient information is available to make a precise adjustment.

Over time, repeated cycles of detection, localization, and correction refine the model. Each iteration reduces the difference between predicted and observed outcomes. The model becomes more stable because its structure more accurately represents the system it is modeling. This stability does not prevent change. It allows change to occur in a controlled manner, where each update improves alignment without introducing new sources of variation.

Feedback integration is the mechanism that prevents drift. It maintains the connection between internal representation and external behavior by ensuring that discrepancies lead to targeted structural updates. The system remains adaptive, but its adaptation is constrained by the requirement that each change improves its ability to map and predict the environment.

Closing the Feedback Loop

A feedback loop closes when the system links an outcome back to the exact process that produced it and updates that process before the next execution. The loop is not complete when an outcome is observed or even when an error is detected. It is complete when the detection, localization, and correction occur within a structure that can be executed again without variation. This restores the system's ability to converge toward alignment because each cycle reduces the same source of error rather than generating new ones.

The loop begins at the point of execution, where an input is transformed through a defined sequence of variables and relationships to produce an output. That sequence must be preserved. If the pathway is not recorded, the system cannot reconnect the outcome to the transformations that generated it. Traceability is therefore a prerequisite for closure. The system must carry forward a representation of each step so that the pathway can be inspected after the result is known.

Outcome measurement must be translated into the same variable structure used during execution. External results are not directly comparable to internal states unless they are represented in a compatible form. This translation aligns the external signal with the internal model, allowing the system to measure deviation as a difference between corresponding variables rather than as a general mismatch. Without this alignment, the system cannot determine what aspect of the output failed.

Detection converts this difference into a structured error. The system identifies which variables do not match expected states and quantifies the direction and magnitude of the deviation. This creates a defined signal that can be traced through the reasoning chain. Detection must occur at a resolution that matches the structure of the model. If it is too coarse, multiple sources of error are combined, and localization becomes ambiguous.

Localization reconnects the error to the first transformation that produced it. The system replays the sequence of transitions, comparing expected intermediate states to those required to produce the observed outcome. The first divergence marks the point where the model no longer reflects the system. This step isolates a single variable definition, relationship condition, or transition rule that must be adjusted. Without this isolation, correction spreads across the model and introduces additional variation.

Correction modifies the identified component and then propagates the change forward through the sequence. The update must be constrained so that it resolves the detected error without altering unrelated pathways. This requires that variables have stable boundaries and that relationships are applied under fixed conditions. When these constraints are present, the system can adjust a specific element and predict how that adjustment will influence subsequent states.

The loop remains open if the corrected process is not used in the next execution. Reintegration ensures that the updated structure replaces the previous version within the system. The same input, when processed again, must move through the modified pathway. If the system reverts to prior patterns or introduces variation in execution, the correction does not accumulate. Each cycle must build on the last, reducing error across repeated instances.

Timing determines whether the loop can be closed effectively. When feedback is delayed, the system must preserve the original pathway until the outcome is observed. This requires storing the sequence and its associated state so that it can be evaluated when the signal arrives. If the system discards or overwrites this information, the connection between action and outcome is lost, and the loop cannot close.

Signal isolation prevents incorrect updates. External outcomes often contain variation that is not related to the variables within the model. The system must filter this noise and extract the portion of the signal that corresponds to the defined structure. If noise is treated as error, the system will modify components that are functioning correctly, creating instability. Accurate closure depends on aligning the feedback signal with the variables and relationships that produced the output.

A closed loop produces cumulative refinement. Each cycle reduces the same class of error because the system corrects the specific transformation that generated it. Over time, the model's structure converges toward the behavior of the environment. The pathway from input to output becomes stable, and repeated execution yields consistent results that align with observed conditions.

Restoring correction requires maintaining every part of this loop. The system must preserve its pathways, translate outcomes into its internal structure, detect and localize error at the correct resolution, apply constrained updates, and reintegrate those updates into future execution. When any part is missing, error persists. When the loop is intact, the system improves through direct interaction with the environment, refining its structure with each cycle.

Updating Models with Data

A model improves when incoming data is translated into structured updates that alter specific components without destabilizing the rest of the system. Data does not refine a model by accumulation alone. It refines a model when each observation is mapped onto existing variables, compared against predicted states, and used to adjust the relationships or constraints that produced the deviation. Continuous refinement is the process of integrating new information in a way that preserves structure while increasing alignment.

The update cycle begins with data ingestion. Observations must be converted into the same variable format used by the model. This requires consistent measurement and representation. If incoming data is encoded differently from internal states, the system cannot perform a direct comparison. Standardized representation ensures that each new observation can be placed into the model as a state that corresponds to a specific configuration of variables.

Comparison follows ingestion. The model generates a predicted state based on its current structure, and this predicted state is compared to the observed state derived from data. The difference between these states is expressed as a deviation across variables. This deviation is not treated as a general mismatch. It is decomposed into specific discrepancies that can be traced back through the model's relationships and transitions.

Localization connects each discrepancy to the transformation that produced it. By tracing the sequence of transitions, the system identifies where the predicted state diverged from the observed state. This may occur at the level of variable definition, where boundaries do not match the system being modeled, or at the level of relationships, where conditions or magnitudes are incorrect. Localization isolates the component that requires adjustment, allowing the update to be targeted rather than distributed across the model.

Adjustment modifies the identified component. This modification must be constrained so that it resolves the detected deviation without introducing new inconsistencies. For a variable, this may involve refining its boundaries or its method of measurement. For a relationship, it may involve adjusting the conditions under which it applies or the magnitude of its effect. The update is applied within the existing architecture, preserving the integrity of other components.

Recalculation propagates the adjustment forward. Once the modification is made, the system re-executes the sequence of transitions from the point of change. This produces a new predicted state, which is again compared to observed data. This iterative process continues until the deviation is reduced to an acceptable level. Each iteration refines the model's structure, improving its ability to generate outputs that align with the environment.

Data weighting controls how updates are applied across multiple observations. Not all data points carry equal relevance. Differences in measurement quality, context, and conditions influence how strongly a particular observation should affect the model. The system must assign weight based on these factors, allowing more reliable data to drive larger adjustments while limiting the influence of noisy or uncertain inputs.

Temporal integration ensures that updates reflect changes over time. Systems evolve, and relationships that were accurate under one set of conditions may shift under another. The model must track when data was collected and how conditions have changed since then. This allows it to distinguish between structural inaccuracies and changes in the system itself. Updates can then be applied in a way that maintains alignment with current conditions while preserving knowledge of past states.

Stability constraints prevent overcorrection. Large adjustments based on limited data can destabilize the model, causing it to oscillate between states rather than converging. The system must limit the magnitude of each update and require consistency across observations before making significant changes. This ensures that refinement proceeds in controlled increments, maintaining the integrity of the model as it evolves.

Accumulation of updates produces convergence. As the system integrates data over repeated cycles, the discrepancies between predicted and observed states decrease. The model's variables, relationships, and constraints become calibrated to the behavior of the system being represented. This convergence is not a static endpoint. It is a dynamic equilibrium where the model continues to adjust as new data is introduced, maintaining alignment over time.

Continuous refinement depends on maintaining the full update loop. Data must be represented consistently, compared at the correct resolution, localized to specific components, and integrated through constrained adjustments. When this loop operates without interruption, the model evolves in a controlled manner, increasing its accuracy while preserving stability. The system does not rely on accumulated information alone. It relies on structured integration, where each piece of data contributes to a precise modification of the architecture that generates its outputs.

Error as Input

A system improves when it treats error as structured information rather than as a signal to suppress or ignore. Error is not a failure state. It is a measurable difference between a predicted state and an observed state. When this difference is captured at the level of variables and relationships, it becomes an input that can be processed in the same way as any other data. The system does not react to error emotionally or heuristically. It incorporates error into its model as a source of correction.

The process begins with representing error in the same format as the model. A deviation must be expressed as a change in variable state, not as a general mismatch. This requires translating the observed outcome into the model's variable structure and subtracting the predicted state from it. The result is a set of differences that specify where and how the model failed. Each difference corresponds to a component within the system, making it possible to trace the error back to its origin.

Once represented, error must be decomposed. A single incorrect output often reflects multiple deviations across different parts of the model. The system separates these into individual discrepancies, each tied to a specific variable or relationship. This prevents the system from applying broad corrections that affect unrelated components. By isolating each deviation, the system can address the underlying cause without introducing additional instability.

Mapping error to structure is the next step. The system traces each discrepancy through the sequence of transitions to identify the first transformation that produced it. This establishes a direct link between the observed error and the structural element responsible. The mapping process converts error from an outcome-level signal into a component-level input, allowing the system to target its updates precisely.

Integration occurs when the mapped error is used to adjust the model. The system modifies the identified variable definition, relationship condition, or transition rule to reduce the discrepancy. This adjustment is constrained so that it resolves the error without altering other pathways that are functioning correctly. The modification is then propagated forward through the model to ensure that it produces a new predicted state that aligns more closely with observed conditions.

Error accumulation provides a pattern over time. Individual discrepancies may reflect noise or transient conditions, but repeated occurrences of similar errors indicate a structural misalignment. The system tracks these patterns, increasing the weight of errors that occur consistently and reducing the influence of isolated deviations. This allows the model to focus its adjustments on persistent sources of error rather than on random variation.

Error must also be contextualized. The same discrepancy may arise under different conditions for different reasons. The system must account for the state of other variables and the context in which the error occurred. This ensures that the adjustment addresses the correct relationship or condition. Without this context, the system may apply a correction that resolves the error in one situation but introduces new errors in another.

Using error as input requires preserving the pathway that generated it. If the system does not maintain a trace of its reasoning process, it cannot connect the error to the specific transformation that produced it. Traceability allows the system to replay the sequence, identify the point of divergence, and apply a targeted update. Without this, error remains at the level of output, and correction becomes approximate.

Error-driven updates must be integrated into future execution. Once a correction is applied, the system must use the updated structure when processing new inputs. This ensures that the adjustment accumulates over time, reducing the likelihood of repeating the same error. If the system reverts to prior patterns or introduces variation in execution, the benefit of the correction is lost.

Treating error as input transforms the role of mistakes within the system. Errors are no longer endpoints that signal failure. They are data points that provide information about the structure of the model. Each error contributes to refining the variables, relationships, and constraints that define the system's behavior. Over time, this process reduces deviation between predicted and observed states, allowing the model to converge toward accurate representation.

A system that processes error structurally maintains alignment through continuous correction. It does not rely on avoiding mistakes. It uses them as part of its operation, integrating each discrepancy into the architecture that generates its outputs. This creates a feedback-driven model where improvement is built into the system's design, and where each cycle of execution contributes to refining its structure.

PART V

DECISION ARCHITECTURE

Chapter 15

What a Decision Is

A decision is the selection of a specific pathway through a structured model that converts a current state into a future state under constraint. It is not a moment of choice in isolation. It is the execution of a defined sequence where variables, relationships, and constraints interact to produce a transition from one configuration of the system to another. The quality of a decision is determined by the structure that generates it, not by the outcome alone. Outcomes are influenced by external variation, but the decision is fully defined by the pathway chosen within the model.

A decision begins with state definition. The system must represent its current configuration in terms of variables that have stable boundaries. This state includes both internal variables and relevant external conditions. Without an accurate representation of the current state, the system cannot evaluate how different pathways will alter that state. The decision process operates on this representation, making it the foundation for all subsequent transformations.

From this state, the system identifies possible transitions. Each transition corresponds to a sequence of relationships that can be applied to move the system from its current configuration to a new one. These transitions are constrained by the model. Not all pathways are valid, and the system must limit its consideration to those that operate within defined conditions. This restriction ensures that the decision is grounded in the structure of the model rather than in unconstrained possibility.

Evaluation of transitions requires projecting how each pathway alters the state. The system applies its relationships in sequence, generating predicted states for each option. These projections are not guesses. They are the result of executing the model under different initial conditions. Each predicted state reflects how the system expects variables to interact if that pathway is chosen.

Constraints then filter these predicted states. Some outcomes may violate boundaries defined within the model, such as exceeding limits on variable states or conflicting with required conditions. These pathways are removed from consideration. The remaining options represent valid transitions that the system can execute without breaking its structure.

Selection occurs when the system chooses one pathway from the remaining set. This choice is based on criteria defined within the model, such as minimizing deviation from a target state, maintaining stability, or optimizing a specific variable. The criteria must be explicit. If selection is based on implicit or shifting criteria, the decision process becomes unstable because the system cannot apply the same evaluation across instances.

Execution follows selection. The system applies the sequence of relationships associated with the chosen pathway, transforming the current state into a new state. This transformation is recorded, preserving the pathway that was taken. This record is necessary for feedback integration, allowing the system to evaluate the decision after its outcome is observed.

A decision is therefore not a single action. It is a structured process that includes state representation, pathway generation, projection, constraint filtering, selection, and execution. Each component must operate within the architecture of the model to ensure that the decision reflects the system's structure.

The distinction between decision and outcome is critical. A decision can be structurally correct even if the outcome is unfavorable due to external variation. Conversely, a decision can be structurally incorrect while producing a favorable outcome by chance. Evaluating decisions requires examining the pathway that generated them, not just the result.

This allows the system to refine its structure based on the validity of its reasoning rather than on isolated outcomes.

Consistency in decision-making arises from the stability of the underlying model. When variables are defined clearly, relationships are applied under fixed conditions, and transitions follow a structured sequence, the system produces decisions that are repeatable given the same inputs. This repeatability allows for refinement through feedback, as the system can identify and correct deviations in its process.

A decision is the point where the model interacts with the environment. It converts internal structure into external action. The quality of that interaction depends on how accurately the model represents the system and how consistently the decision process applies that representation. By defining decisions as structured pathways, the system maintains control over how it moves from one state to another, ensuring that each action is grounded in the architecture that governs its behavior.

Decisions as Output of Structure

A decision is the direct result of how a system is built. It does not originate at the moment of choice. It emerges from the configuration of variables, the relationships that connect them, and the constraints that limit how they can change. When a system produces a decision, it is executing its architecture. The output reflects the structure that processed the input, not a separate act layered on top of it.

The pathway to a decision begins before any explicit evaluation occurs. Variable definitions determine what the system can see. If critical components are excluded or boundaries are unstable, the system constructs an incomplete state. Every subsequent transformation operates on this state. The decision that emerges cannot account for what was never represented. It follows the structure that was available at the start of the process.

Relationships then shape how that state evolves. Each interaction between variables directs the flow of change, moving the system toward specific configurations while excluding others. These interactions are applied under defined conditions, and their cumulative effect determines which outcomes become reachable. The decision is not chosen from an unrestricted set of possibilities. It is the endpoint of the pathways that remain valid after these relationships are applied.

Constraint enforcement further limits the system. Boundaries on variables and conditions on relationships remove pathways that violate the model. This restriction narrows the set of possible outcomes before any selection occurs. By the time the system reaches the point of choosing, many options have already been eliminated by the structure itself. The decision is therefore shaped long before it appears as a discrete event.

Selection is often interpreted as the core of decision-making, but within a structured system it is a final step that operates on a constrained set of states. The system evaluates the remaining options based on defined criteria, but these options exist only because the preceding structure allowed them to persist. Changing the structure changes the set of available outcomes, which changes the decision even if the selection criteria remain the same.

Execution completes the process by applying the sequence of transformations associated with the chosen pathway. This step converts the internal state into an external action or outcome. The execution does not redefine the decision. It carries forward the result of the structured process that produced it. The pathway remains traceable from input to output, linking the decision to the architecture that generated it.

Treating decisions as isolated events removes visibility into this process. It focuses attention on the moment of selection while ignoring the structure that determined which options were available and how they were evaluated. This leads to incorrect conclusions about why decisions occur, because the analysis is disconnected from the variables and relationships that produced them.

When decisions are understood as outputs of structure, improvement shifts to the level of the model. Refinement involves adjusting variable definitions, correcting relationships, and enforcing constraints more precisely. These changes alter the pathways that the system can generate, which in turn changes the decisions it produces. The system does not attempt to make better decisions directly. It modifies the architecture that generates them.

Consistency in decisions emerges from stability in structure. When the same input is processed through the same defined sequence of transformations, the resulting decision is repeatable. Variability in decisions arises when the structure changes between instances, either through shifting variable definitions, inconsistent application of relationships, or variation in constraints. Stabilizing these elements stabilizes the outputs.

A decision is therefore not an independent act. It is the visible result of an internal process that begins with representation and ends with execution. By focusing on the structure that produces decisions, the system gains control over its outputs. Each decision becomes a reflection of the architecture, allowing it to be traced, evaluated, and improved through changes to the underlying model rather than through isolated adjustments at the point of choice.

Inputs, Models, Outputs

A decision pipeline is the structured flow that converts external information into a defined action through a model that enforces how that information is processed. It is not a sequence of loosely connected steps. It is a continuous system where each stage constrains the next. Inputs are transformed into variables, variables are processed through relationships within the model, and the resulting state produces an output that reflects the structure of the system. When the pipeline is stable, the same input produces the same pathway and therefore the same class of output.

The pipeline begins with input acquisition and filtration. Raw information enters the system with varying levels of relevance and noise. The system must isolate the portion of the input that corresponds to its defined variables. This requires filtering out signals that do not map onto the model and resolving ambiguity before integration. If irrelevant or misinterpreted inputs are allowed into the system, they alter the initial state and propagate error through the entire pipeline. The accuracy of the output is therefore constrained by the precision of this first stage.

Input translation converts filtered information into variables with defined boundaries. Each element of the input must be assigned to a variable that maintains identity across the reasoning process. This step standardizes representation, ensuring that different instances of similar inputs produce the same internal structure. Without consistent translation, the system begins each execution from a different configuration, making repeatability impossible. The model does not process raw inputs. It processes structured variables derived from those inputs.

The model stage applies relationships to these variables. Interactions are executed under defined conditions, and each transformation produces a new state. This stage is the core of the pipeline. It determines how changes in one variable propagate through the system and how multiple variables combine to produce effects. The sequence of transformations must be explicit and ordered. Each step depends on the state produced by the previous one, creating a continuous chain from input to output.

Constraint enforcement operates within the model stage. At each transformation, the system verifies that variables remain within their boundaries and that relationships are applied only under valid conditions. This prevents the pipeline from entering states that violate the structure of the model. Constraints reduce the number of possible pathways, ensuring that the system operates within a defined space where outputs remain aligned with the architecture.

Intermediate state tracking maintains continuity across the pipeline. After each transformation, the system records the current state of all variables. This allows the pipeline to be inspected and ensures that subsequent transformations operate on the correct inputs. It also enables feedback integration, where the system can trace back through these states to identify where deviations occurred when comparing outputs to observed outcomes.

The output stage converts the final internal state into an external action or conclusion. This conversion must preserve the structure of the state, ensuring that the output reflects the variables and relationships that produced it. The output is not an independent decision. It is the endpoint of the pipeline, carrying forward the result of all prior transformations.

Feedback integration closes the pipeline by linking the output back to the input through the model. Observed outcomes are translated into the same variable structure and compared to the predicted state. Differences are traced back through the pipeline to identify where the model deviated. Corrections are applied at the point of divergence, and the updated structure is used in subsequent executions. This creates a cycle where each pass through the pipeline refines the model.

Stability in the pipeline requires that each stage operates consistently. Input translation must produce the same variable structure for the same information. The model must apply relationships in a fixed sequence with defined conditions. Constraints must be enforced without variation. Output conversion must preserve the structure of the final state. When these elements are stable, the pipeline produces repeatable outputs and can be refined through feedback.

A breakdown at any stage disrupts the entire system. Inconsistent input translation alters the initial state. Variable drift changes how relationships are applied. Missing constraints allow invalid states to propagate. Loss of intermediate tracking prevents localization of error. Each failure introduces variation that compounds as the pipeline progresses, leading to outputs that cannot be traced back to a consistent structure.

The decision pipeline organizes reasoning into a controlled flow. Inputs are not interpreted in isolation. They are transformed into a structured representation, processed through a defined model, and converted into outputs that reflect that process. By maintaining stability across each stage, the system ensures that decisions are generated through a repeatable pathway that can be inspected, corrected, and refined over time.

Defining the Problem Correctly

A system can only produce a valid output if the problem it is solving is represented with the correct structure. Problem framing determines which variables are included, how they are bounded, and what relationships are considered relevant. It establishes the initial state on which the entire decision pipeline operates. If the framing is incorrect, every subsequent transformation applies to a distorted representation. The system may execute its model accurately, but the output will reflect the structure of the framing rather than the structure of the actual problem.

Framing begins with identifying the target state. The system must define what constitutes resolution in terms of variable configurations. This is not a general objective. It is a specific arrangement of variables that the system aims to produce or maintain. Without a defined target state, the model cannot evaluate whether a pathway moves the system toward or away from resolution. The absence of this definition leads to outputs that are internally consistent but directionless.

The next step is boundary definition. The system must determine which components belong inside the problem and which remain external. These boundaries define the scope of the model. Including irrelevant components increases complexity without improving accuracy, while excluding relevant ones removes critical pathways that influence the outcome. Boundaries must align with how the underlying system is organized so that interactions are represented correctly.

Variable selection follows boundary definition. The system identifies components within the defined scope that can change state and influence the outcome. Each variable must have stable boundaries and a representation that allows relationships to be applied consistently. If variables are too broad, distinct effects are merged and cannot be separated. If they are too narrow, the system becomes fragmented and difficult to process. The chosen variables determine what the model can detect and manipulate.

Relationship inclusion determines how variables interact within the frame. The system must map only those interactions that operate within the defined boundaries and influence the target state. Including relationships that do not apply introduces noise, while excluding relevant ones removes pathways that drive change. The set of relationships defines how the system can move from its current state toward the target.

Constraint definition limits the set of valid states and transitions. Constraints establish what configurations are possible within the frame and prevent the system from generating outcomes that violate the structure of the problem. These constraints may arise from physical limits, logical rules, or contextual conditions. By enforcing them, the system ensures that its reasoning remains grounded in the conditions that define the problem.

Temporal framing determines how changes unfold. The system must account for the sequence and timing of interactions, specifying whether effects occur immediately or over delayed intervals. Without this, the model collapses dynamic processes into static relationships, producing outputs that do not reflect how the system evolves. Temporal structure allows the system to represent progression from the current state to the target state through a series of transitions.

Framing must also address uncertainty. Not all variables or relationships will be fully specified at the outset. The system must define how to handle incomplete information, whether by assigning provisional states, maintaining ranges, or deferring certain transitions. These methods must be part of the frame, ensuring that uncertainty is managed consistently rather than resolved through uncontrolled inference.

Incorrect framing often appears as a mismatch between outputs and observed outcomes that persists despite repeated adjustments to the model. In these cases, the issue is not within the relationships or transitions. It is within the initial representation. The system is solving a different problem than the one it intends to solve. Recognizing this requires stepping back to the framing stage and redefining variables, boundaries, or constraints so that the model aligns with the actual structure of the problem.

A correct frame produces a model where variables correspond to real components, relationships reflect actual interactions, and constraints match the conditions of the system. The decision pipeline then operates on a representation that can generate outputs aligned with reality. Each transformation within the model builds on a structure that accurately captures what matters.

Problem framing is therefore the point where reasoning either aligns with the system or diverges from it. It defines the architecture within which all processing occurs. When the frame is constructed correctly, the system can apply its model with confidence that its outputs reflect the problem it is meant to solve. When it is not, no level of refinement within the model can compensate for the misalignment introduced at the start.

Chapter 16

Decision Mechanics

A decision is executed when the system applies its model to move from a defined current state to a selected future state through a constrained sequence of transformations. Decision mechanics describe how this execution occurs at the level of variables, relationships, and transitions. It is the operational layer where the structure of the model is applied in real time. When these mechanics are stable, the system produces decisions that are consistent with its architecture. When they are not, the system introduces variation during execution, and outputs no longer reflect the model that is supposed to generate them.

The process begins with state initialization. The system constructs a representation of the current configuration using its defined variables. This state must be complete enough to support the relationships that will be applied. Missing or misrepresented variables alter the initial conditions, which changes how subsequent transformations unfold. Decision mechanics depend on the accuracy of this starting state because every transition is applied relative to it.

Once the state is defined, the system activates the relevant subset of relationships. Not all interactions in the model apply to every decision. The system must identify which relationships are valid under the current conditions and bring them into the active set. This activation is determined by the state of the variables and the constraints defined within the model. Incorrect activation introduces relationships that do not apply or omits those that do, distorting the pathway from the outset.

Transition sequencing then determines how these relationships are applied. Each step in the sequence represents a transformation that moves the system from one state to another. The order of these steps is not arbitrary. Relationships often depend on the outputs of prior transformations, and altering the sequence changes intermediate states. Decision mechanics enforce a defined order, ensuring that each transformation operates on the correct inputs.

At each transition, the system applies a relationship to the current state, producing a new configuration of variables. This application must preserve the identity of each variable and adhere to the conditions that define the relationship. The transformation is not approximate. It follows the defined rules of the model. This precision ensures that the pathway remains aligned with the structure that generated it.

Constraint checks are performed at every stage. After each transformation, the system verifies that the new state does not violate the boundaries of any variable and that all relationships have been applied under valid conditions. If a violation is detected, the pathway is invalidated or corrected before proceeding. This prevents the decision process from entering states that are inconsistent with the model.

Parallel pathways may be evaluated during this process. The system can simulate multiple sequences of transformations, each representing a different potential decision. These pathways are generated by applying different combinations of relationships or by altering initial conditions within allowable bounds. Each pathway produces a projected state, which is then evaluated against the system's criteria for selection.

Selection occurs when the system chooses one pathway from the set of valid options. This choice is based on defined criteria, such as minimizing deviation from a target state or maintaining stability across variables. The criteria must be consistent across decisions. If they shift between instances, the system introduces variability that is not accounted for by the model.

Execution applies the selected sequence of transformations to the current state, producing the final state that defines the decision. This state is then converted into an external action or conclusion. The execution process preserves the pathway, allowing it to be traced and evaluated after the outcome is observed.

Timing influences how these mechanics operate. Some transformations occur immediately, while others introduce delays. The system must account for these temporal differences, ensuring that relationships are applied at the correct point in the sequence. Ignoring timing collapses the process into a single step, removing the ability to track how changes accumulate and interact over time.

Decision mechanics also require stability under varying conditions. The same input must activate the same relationships, follow the same sequence, and apply the same transformations. This repeatability ensures that the decision reflects the model rather than variation in execution. When mechanics are stable, differences in decisions arise from differences in input or structure, not from inconsistencies in how the process is carried out.

A decision is therefore the result of executing a defined sequence within a structured system. The mechanics that govern this execution determine whether the output remains aligned with the model. By stabilizing these mechanics, the system ensures that each decision is produced through a pathway that can be traced, evaluated, and refined, maintaining consistency across instances and enabling continuous improvement through feedback.

Constraints and Tradeoffs

A system operates within limits that define what states are possible and what transitions can occur between them. Constraints establish these limits. They define the boundaries of variables, the conditions under which relationships apply, and the range of outcomes the system can produce. Tradeoffs emerge from these constraints. When the system selects one pathway, it excludes others because the structure does not allow all outcomes to be achieved simultaneously. Decisions are therefore shaped by the boundaries of the system, not by unrestricted choice.

Constraints begin at the level of variables. Each variable has a defined range of valid states. These ranges are not arbitrary. They reflect the conditions under which the system can operate without breaking its structure. When a variable approaches its boundary, the set of valid transitions narrows. Certain relationships may no longer apply, and others may become dominant. This changes the pathways available to the system, altering how it can move from its current state to a future one.

Relationships also impose constraints. Each interaction operates only under specific conditions. These conditions limit when and how variables can influence one another. If the conditions are not met, the relationship is inactive, and the pathway it would create is removed from consideration. This restriction ensures that the system does not apply transformations that are not valid within its structure. It also means that the availability of certain pathways depends on the current state of the system.

Constraints accumulate across the model. Variable boundaries and relationship conditions combine to form a space of valid states and transitions. Within this space, the system can operate freely. Outside it, transitions are not allowed. This space defines the feasible set of outcomes. Any decision must result in a state that lies within these boundaries. The system cannot produce an outcome that violates them without breaking its structure.

Tradeoffs arise because constraints limit what can be achieved simultaneously. When the system moves toward one region of the valid state space, it often moves away from another. This is not a conflict introduced by preference. It is a structural consequence of the model. Variables and relationships interact in ways that make certain combinations of states incompatible. The system must therefore select which direction to move, knowing that other directions become less accessible.

Evaluation of tradeoffs requires projecting how different pathways alter the state of the system within these constraints. Each pathway leads to a different configuration of variables, and each configuration satisfies some conditions while approaching or reaching the boundaries of others. The system must compare these configurations based on its criteria, understanding that improving one aspect may degrade another because of the underlying constraints.

Temporal factors influence tradeoffs as well. Some constraints are immediate, while others emerge over time. A pathway that appears valid in the short term may lead to boundary violations in later states. The system must account for how constraints evolve as transitions are applied, ensuring that the selected pathway remains within the valid space throughout its execution.

Hidden constraints introduce additional complexity. These are limits that affect the system but are not explicitly represented in the model. Their presence is often detected when predicted pathways lead to outcomes that are not achievable in practice. Identifying and incorporating these constraints into the model reduces discrepancies between predicted and observed behavior, improving alignment.

Constraint prioritization determines how the system resolves conflicts between competing limits. Some constraints are absolute and cannot be violated, while others are flexible within a range. The model must define which constraints take precedence when tradeoffs occur. This prioritization guides the selection process, ensuring that the system maintains critical boundaries while optimizing within the remaining space.

Tradeoffs are therefore not subjective compromises. They are the result of operating within a structured system where constraints define what is possible. The system does not choose between arbitrary options. It selects pathways that navigate the boundaries imposed by its variables and relationships. Understanding these boundaries allows the system to make decisions that remain aligned with its structure, avoiding transitions that would lead to invalid or unstable states.

By mapping constraints explicitly and evaluating tradeoffs within that map, the system gains control over its decision space. It can predict which pathways are feasible, which lead to boundary conditions, and how different choices interact with the limits of the model. This transforms decision-making from an open-ended selection into a constrained optimization within a defined structure, where each choice reflects the architecture that governs the system.

Scenario Simulation

A system reduces uncertainty by running its model forward before committing to a pathway. Scenario simulation applies the same variables, relationships, constraints, and sequencing used in execution, but it does so in a contained loop that generates projected states rather than external actions. The purpose is not to predict a single outcome. It is to map how different initial choices propagate through the structure and where each pathway encounters constraints, amplification, or instability. When simulation is built on the same architecture as execution, the projected states reflect how the system will behave once the decision is applied.

The process begins with state cloning. The current configuration of variables is duplicated so that multiple pathways can be explored without altering the live state. This clone must preserve all relevant variables and their boundaries. If the cloned state omits elements or alters representation, the simulation diverges before any transformation occurs. Each scenario starts from the same baseline, allowing differences in outcomes to be attributed to differences in the applied pathway rather than to variation in initial conditions.

Pathway generation follows. The system constructs candidate sequences by activating different subsets of relationships or by altering controllable inputs within allowed ranges. These pathways are not arbitrary. They must remain within the model's constraints and follow valid sequencing rules. Each candidate represents a decision option encoded as a sequence of transformations that can be executed step by step.

Simulation then applies transitions in order. For each candidate pathway, the system runs the same transformation sequence it would use during execution, producing a series of intermediate states. Each transition operates under its defined conditions, preserving variable identity and enforcing constraints. The result is a trajectory through the model's state space, showing how the system evolves from the initial configuration to a projected future state.

Constraint interaction becomes visible during this process. As variables move through their ranges, some pathways encounter boundaries earlier than others. Certain relationships deactivate when conditions are no longer met, while others become dominant. These interactions change the direction and magnitude of subsequent transformations. Simulation reveals where pathways narrow, stall, or produce unstable configurations, allowing the system to eliminate options that would fail during execution.

Temporal structure is preserved within each scenario. Relationships that operate with delay are applied at the appropriate stage in the sequence, allowing the system to observe how effects accumulate over time. This prevents the model from compressing dynamic behavior into a single step. The trajectory shows not only the final state but also the sequence of intermediate states that lead to it, which is critical for identifying points of instability or divergence.

Parallel evaluation compares the resulting trajectories. Each scenario produces a final state along with a pathway that can be inspected. The system evaluates these states against its defined criteria, such as maintaining variable stability, remaining within constraint boundaries, or moving toward a target configuration. Because each scenario follows the same structural rules, differences in outcome can be attributed to the pathway itself rather than to variation in processing.

Sensitivity analysis extends the simulation by introducing controlled variation in inputs or parameters. Small changes are applied to the initial state or to specific relationships to observe how the trajectory shifts. This reveals how dependent each pathway is on precise conditions. Pathways that remain stable under variation are more robust. Those that diverge rapidly indicate regions of the model where small deviations produce large effects.

Simulation must remain coupled to the execution model. If the system uses different rules or compressed transitions during simulation, the projected states will not match what occurs during actual execution. The same variables, relationships, sequencing, and constraint checks must be applied. This ensures that the simulation is a direct preview of how the decision will unfold when enacted.

Resource limits constrain how many scenarios can be evaluated. The system must balance depth and breadth, deciding how many pathways to simulate and how far forward to project each one. This selection is itself structured. Pathways that violate constraints early can be terminated, allowing resources to be allocated to those that remain viable. The system focuses on exploring regions of the state space that are reachable and relevant to the decision.

Scenario simulation transforms decision-making from reactive selection into controlled projection. By pre-executing pathways within the model, the system identifies which sequences lead to stable and valid states before committing to action. This reduces the likelihood of entering configurations that require correction after execution. The decision that is ultimately selected is therefore not chosen in isolation. It is the result of evaluating multiple structured trajectories and selecting the one that remains aligned with the system's constraints and objectives across its full sequence of transformations.

Probability and Uncertainty

A decision system rarely operates with full specification of all variables and relationships. Uncertainty enters when parts of the state are unknown, when measurements carry error, or when relationships change across conditions. Probability is the mechanism that allows the system to continue operating under these conditions by representing unknowns as distributions rather than fixed values. This does not replace structure. It extends the model so that each transformation can operate on ranges of possible states instead of single points.

Uncertainty begins at the level of variables. When a variable cannot be assigned a precise state, the system represents it as a distribution over possible values. This distribution must be bounded and defined in the same space as the variable itself. It encodes what is known about the variable and what remains unresolved. Each possible state carries a weight that reflects how consistent it is with available information. The system does not collapse this distribution prematurely. It carries it forward through the model so that relationships can act on the full range of possibilities.

Relationships must then operate on these distributions. A transformation applied to an uncertain variable produces a new distribution for the target variable. The form of this transformation depends on how the relationship behaves across the range of inputs. Linear interactions propagate uncertainty in a predictable way, while nonlinear interactions can amplify or compress it. The system must apply the same conditional rules used in deterministic processing, but it must do so across the entire distribution rather than at a single value. This produces a set of possible outcomes, each with an associated weight.

State representation expands to include uncertainty across all variables. At any point in the sequence, the system holds a joint distribution that describes the possible configurations of the system and their relative likelihoods. This representation allows the system to project how uncertainty evolves as transitions are applied. Some pathways reduce uncertainty by constraining variables, while others increase it by introducing additional variation. The system tracks these changes as part of the state.

Decision evaluation under uncertainty requires comparing distributions rather than single outcomes. Each candidate pathway produces a distribution of possible final states. The system evaluates these distributions based on criteria that account for both expected outcomes and variability. A pathway that produces a favorable average state but with high variance may be less desirable than one with a slightly lower average but greater stability. The evaluation criteria must therefore incorporate both central tendency and dispersion.

Constraint interaction remains active under uncertainty. Some portions of a distribution may fall outside valid boundaries, while others remain within them. The system must determine how to handle these cases. It may truncate invalid regions, redistribute probability mass, or eliminate pathways where a significant portion of outcomes violate constraints. This ensures that decisions remain grounded within the feasible state space even when inputs are incomplete.

Temporal structure influences how uncertainty propagates. Early-stage uncertainty can expand or contract as relationships are applied. Delayed interactions may introduce new sources of variation at later stages in the sequence. The system must track how distributions evolve over time, allowing it to identify points where uncertainty becomes dominant and where additional information would most improve alignment.

Information acquisition becomes part of the decision process. When uncertainty significantly affects the outcome, the system can allocate resources to reduce it before executing a pathway. This involves identifying which variables contribute most to outcome variability and obtaining data that refines their distributions. The system integrates this new information into the model, narrowing the range of possible states and improving the precision of its projections.

Calibration ensures that the system's representation of uncertainty matches observed behavior. If the model assigns too much weight to unlikely states or too little to common ones, its decisions will be misaligned. Calibration is achieved through feedback, where predicted distributions are compared to observed outcomes and adjusted accordingly. This process refines how the system represents uncertainty over time.

Decision-making under incomplete information does not eliminate uncertainty. It structures it. The system maintains a representation of what is known and what is not, applies its model across this representation, and selects pathways based on how distributions of outcomes align with its criteria and constraints. This allows the system to operate in environments where full information is not available, while preserving the integrity of its structure and maintaining the ability to refine its model as new data is introduced.

Chapter 17

Execution and Iteration

A system moves from decision to outcome by executing a defined pathway and then re-entering the model with the resulting state. Execution converts internal structure into external change. Iteration reconnects that change to the model so that subsequent decisions operate on an updated representation. These two processes are not separate phases. They form a continuous cycle where each execution produces the conditions for the next iteration. When this cycle is stable, the system maintains alignment as it operates over time.

Execution begins with committing to a selected pathway. The system takes the sequence of transformations defined during decision mechanics and applies them to the current state. Each transformation must be executed under the same conditions used during evaluation. If execution alters the sequence, skips steps, or introduces new relationships, the outcome will diverge from the projected state. Consistency between simulation and execution is required for the model to remain predictive.

State transition during execution occurs in the external system. Variables within the model correspond to components in the environment, and applying a transformation changes their external configuration. These changes may occur immediately or unfold over time, depending on the temporal structure of the relationships. The system must track these transitions as they occur, maintaining a representation of how the state evolves after execution.

Observation captures the resulting state. The system measures the external configuration after the pathway has been applied and translates it back into its variable structure. This translation must preserve the boundaries and definitions used within the model so that the observed state can be compared directly to the predicted state. Without consistent representation, the system cannot determine whether the execution aligned with its expectations.

Deviation emerges when the observed state differs from the predicted state. This difference reflects either external variation or a misalignment within the model. The system expresses this deviation in terms of variable differences, creating a structured signal that can be traced back through the executed pathway. This signal is the entry point for iteration.

Iteration begins with localization of the deviation. The system traces the executed sequence to identify where the actual transition diverged from the modeled transformation. This may occur because a relationship was mis-specified, because a variable boundary did not match the external system, or because an unmodeled factor influenced the outcome. Identifying the first point of divergence isolates the component that requires adjustment.

Adjustment modifies the model at that point. The system refines the variable definition, updates the conditions of the relationship, or incorporates a new constraint that accounts for the observed behavior. This change is applied within the existing architecture, preserving the structure of other components. After the modification, the system recalculates the pathway to ensure that the updated model produces a state that aligns more closely with observation.

Reintegration places the updated model back into operation. The next execution uses the modified structure, allowing the system to test whether the adjustment reduces deviation. This creates a feedback loop where each iteration builds on the previous one, progressively aligning the model with the behavior of the environment.

Iteration also operates across multiple executions. Patterns of deviation that appear consistently indicate structural issues within the model. The system aggregates these patterns, increasing the weight of adjustments that address persistent discrepancies. This prevents overcorrection based on isolated observations and ensures that refinement is driven by stable signals.

Temporal continuity is maintained across iterations. The state resulting from one execution becomes the starting point for the next decision. This creates a chain of states that evolves over time, allowing the system to operate in dynamic environments where conditions change. Each iteration updates the model while preserving the continuity of the system's operation.

Execution without iteration leads to drift. The system continues to apply its model, but discrepancies accumulate because they are not used to refine the structure. Iteration without consistent execution leads to instability, as updates are applied to a model that is not being executed in a controlled manner. The combination of both processes ensures that the system remains both active and aligned.

Execution and iteration together form the operational core of a structured system. Decisions are not endpoints. They are transitions within a continuous cycle where each action generates information that feeds back into the model. By maintaining consistency in execution and precision in iteration, the system ensures that its structure evolves in response to real conditions while preserving the integrity of its decision-making process.

Action as Model Testing

A system does not validate its model through internal consistency. It validates it through action. Every executed decision is a test of whether the model's variables, relationships, and constraints correspond to how the external system behaves. Action exposes the model to conditions it cannot fully simulate, forcing a comparison between predicted states and observed outcomes. This comparison generates the signal required to refine the structure.

Execution defines the test conditions. The system selects a pathway and applies it to the current state, producing a sequence of external changes. These changes must be traceable to the internal model. The pathway used during execution is preserved so that the outcome can be linked back to the specific transformations that produced it. Without this trace, the system observes results without knowing how they were generated, which prevents targeted correction.

Observation captures the resulting state after the action is applied. The system measures how variables in the environment have changed and translates those measurements into its internal representation. This translation must align with the model's variable definitions. If the mapping is inconsistent, the system compares incompatible states and misinterprets the result of the test.

Comparison evaluates the difference between the predicted and observed states. The model produces an expected configuration based on the executed pathway. The observed configuration reflects how the system actually responded. The difference between these two states is expressed as a structured deviation across variables. This deviation indicates where the model's representation does not match the external system.

Localization traces this deviation back through the executed sequence. The system identifies the first transformation where the predicted change did not match the observed change. This step isolates the component of the model that failed to represent the system accurately. The error is no longer an abstract mismatch. It is tied to a specific variable definition, relationship condition, or constraint.

Adjustment modifies the identified component. The system refines the structure so that the same transformation, when applied again, produces a state closer to the observed outcome. This adjustment must be constrained to avoid altering unrelated parts of the model. The goal is to correct the pathway at the point of divergence, not to reshape the entire structure.

Re-execution provides validation of the adjustment. The system applies the updated pathway under similar conditions and observes whether the deviation is reduced. If the adjustment is correct, the predicted and observed states converge. If not, the process repeats, further refining the model. Each cycle of action and feedback improves alignment between the model and the system it represents.

Action also reveals unmodeled variables. When repeated deviations occur that cannot be localized within the existing structure, the system must identify factors that are influencing the outcome but are not represented. These variables are incorporated into the model, expanding its scope and increasing its ability to capture the behavior of the environment.

Test conditions influence the quality of feedback. If actions are taken under highly variable or noisy conditions, the resulting observations may not clearly reflect the effect of the pathway. The system must either control conditions to isolate variables or account for variability within its model. This ensures that the feedback signal corresponds to the structure being tested.

Action as testing transforms decision-making into an experimental process. Each decision is not only a means of producing an outcome but also a mechanism for gathering information about the accuracy of the model. The system uses this information to refine its structure, improving its ability to generate outputs that align with reality.

A system that does not treat action as testing cannot maintain alignment. It operates on assumptions that are never validated, allowing discrepancies to accumulate. By integrating action and feedback, the system ensures that every execution contributes to the refinement of its model, maintaining a continuous connection between internal structure and external behavior.

Iterative Refinement

A system improves when each execution cycle produces a targeted update to the structure that generated its output. Iterative refinement is the controlled repetition of this cycle, where the model is adjusted in response to measured deviations and then re-executed under the same architecture. Improvement does not occur through accumulation of experience alone. It occurs when each cycle modifies variables, relationships, or constraints in a way that reduces future error without introducing new instability.

The cycle begins with a defined execution pathway. The system applies its current model to move from the present state to a new state. This pathway must be preserved in detail so that its transformations can be inspected after the outcome is observed. Without a recorded sequence, the system cannot connect results back to the structure that produced them, and refinement becomes diffuse.

Observation captures the resulting state and translates it into the model's variable structure. This translation must maintain consistency with how variables are defined internally. The observed state is then compared to the predicted state generated during execution. The difference between these states is expressed as a set of deviations across variables, forming the signal that drives refinement.

Localization isolates the first transformation in the pathway where the predicted and observed states diverge. This step identifies the specific component of the model that requires adjustment. The system does not modify the entire pathway. It targets the variable definition, relationship condition, or constraint that produced the deviation. This precision prevents the introduction of unnecessary variation into parts of the model that are already aligned.

Adjustment modifies the identified component. The change is constrained so that it resolves the detected deviation while preserving the integrity of other pathways. The system applies the modification and recalculates the sequence from that point forward, producing an updated predicted state. This ensures that the adjustment integrates coherently into the model rather than creating discontinuities.

Re-execution tests the adjustment. The system applies the updated model to a new instance or to a repeated condition, observing whether the deviation is reduced. This step confirms whether the modification improved alignment. If the deviation persists or new discrepancies appear, the cycle repeats, refining the adjustment further.

Accumulation across cycles produces convergence. Repeated corrections to the same class of error reduce its frequency and magnitude. The model becomes calibrated to the behavior of the environment, with variables and relationships adjusted to reflect observed interactions. This convergence is gradual and controlled, avoiding large shifts that could destabilize the system.

Stability constraints regulate the rate of change. Adjustments are applied incrementally, and the system requires consistency across multiple observations before making significant modifications. This prevents overcorrection based on noise or isolated events. The model evolves in a way that preserves continuity, allowing each update to build on previous ones.

Parallel refinement may occur across different parts of the model. Independent pathways can be adjusted simultaneously if their deviations are localized to separate components. The system maintains separation between these updates, ensuring that changes in one area do not introduce unintended effects in another. This allows the model to scale its refinement process without losing control over its structure.

Temporal continuity links each cycle to the next. The state produced by one execution becomes the starting point for the next decision, and the updated model is applied to this new state. This creates a continuous progression where both the system's state and its structure evolve together. Each iteration reflects both the current conditions and the accumulated refinements of prior cycles.

Iterative refinement transforms improvement into a built-in function of the system. Rather than attempting to eliminate error entirely, the system uses each occurrence of error to adjust its structure. Over time, this process reduces deviation between predicted and observed states, allowing the model to operate with increasing accuracy and stability. Continuous improvement is not achieved by isolated changes. It is achieved through a repeated, structured cycle where each execution contributes to the refinement of the architecture that produces it.

Decision Speed vs Accuracy Balance

A decision system operates under finite time, energy, and information. Speed and accuracy are not independent objectives. They are coupled through the structure of the model and the depth at which that structure is executed. Increasing speed reduces the number of variables resolved, the number of transitions evaluated, and the degree of constraint enforcement applied at each step. Increasing accuracy requires expanding those same elements, which increases processing time. The balance is determined by how the system allocates its resources across the pipeline while preserving the integrity of its structure.

Speed emerges from compression. The system reduces the number of explicit transitions by grouping multiple transformations into a single step, limits the resolution of variables, and narrows the set of pathways it evaluates. This reduces processing time but introduces approximation. When compression is applied without control, relationships are executed with incomplete conditions, and variable boundaries become less precise. The pathway remains functional, but it no longer reflects the full structure of the model. The output is generated faster, but it carries increased deviation from what a fully resolved process would produce.

Accuracy emerges from resolution. The system expands variables to their defined boundaries, applies relationships under full conditional checks, and preserves each transition in sequence. It evaluates multiple pathways and tracks intermediate states to ensure that constraints are enforced at every stage. This produces outputs that align closely with the model, but it increases the number of operations required. The system must process more information and maintain more state, which reduces throughput.

The balance between speed and accuracy is not fixed. It is adjusted based on the structure of the problem and the cost of error. When constraints are tight and deviations produce large downstream effects, the system must operate at higher resolution. This ensures that each transformation is valid and that the pathway remains within the feasible state space. When constraints are loose and deviations have limited impact, the system can operate with greater compression, accepting reduced precision in exchange for increased throughput.

Selective resolution allows the system to allocate accuracy where it matters. Not all variables and relationships contribute equally to the outcome. The system identifies components with the highest influence on the final state and applies full resolution to those elements while compressing others. This preserves accuracy in critical pathways while reducing the overall processing load. The model remains structured, but its execution is prioritized according to impact.

Adaptive sequencing adjusts the depth of processing during execution. The system may begin with a compressed evaluation to eliminate clearly invalid pathways and then increase resolution on the remaining options. This staged approach allows the system to reduce the search space quickly and then apply precision where it is most needed. It maintains control over both speed and accuracy by separating coarse filtering from fine evaluation.

Constraint enforcement acts as a safeguard against excessive compression. Even when operating at higher speed, the system must ensure that variable boundaries and relationship conditions are not violated. This limits how much compression can be applied without destabilizing the model. If constraints are ignored, the system may produce outputs quickly, but those outputs may fall outside the valid state space, requiring correction after execution.

Feedback integration calibrates the balance over time. By comparing predicted and observed outcomes, the system identifies where compression introduces unacceptable deviation. It can then increase resolution in those areas while maintaining speed in others. This iterative adjustment aligns the balance with the actual behavior of the system, ensuring that throughput is optimized without sacrificing alignment.

Resource constraints define the operating point. Available time, computational capacity, and information determine how much resolution the system can apply. The model must operate within these limits while maintaining structural integrity. This requires explicit control over how resources are allocated across the pipeline, ensuring that critical components receive sufficient processing while less critical ones are simplified.

The balance between speed and accuracy is therefore a function of structure, constraints, and resource allocation. It is not achieved by choosing one objective over the other. It is achieved by designing the decision process so that compression and resolution are applied in a controlled manner, preserving the pathways that determine alignment while reducing unnecessary computation.

A system that manages this balance maintains both efficiency and reliability. It produces decisions at a rate that matches its operational requirements while ensuring that those decisions remain grounded in the structure of its model. Through continuous feedback and adjustment, the system refines this balance, aligning throughput with the level of precision required by the conditions in which it operates.

PART VI

LEVERAGE AND VALUE CREATION

Chapter 18

Logic as Leverage

A system gains leverage when a small set of structured operations produces consistent effects across a wide range of inputs. Logic provides this leverage by constraining how variables are transformed, ensuring that each step in the reasoning process preserves alignment with the model. When logic is embedded at the level of structure, it reduces the need for repeated reconstruction of decisions. The same defined pathways can be applied across different conditions, producing outputs that remain consistent because the underlying transformations do not change.

Leverage begins with stability in variable definition. When variables maintain fixed boundaries, the system can reuse them across multiple contexts without reinterpretation. This allows relationships to operate on a consistent set of elements, reducing the need to rebuild the representation for each new input. The system invests once in defining the structure and then applies that structure repeatedly. This reuse is the first source of leverage, as it converts effort spent on definition into repeated application.

Relationships amplify this effect. Each defined interaction encodes how changes propagate between variables. Once specified, these interactions can be applied across any state where their conditions are met. The system does not need to derive these relationships each time. It executes them as part of its architecture. This allows a single defined relationship to influence many different pathways, extending its impact beyond a single instance.

Constraint enforcement further increases leverage by reducing the number of pathways the system must consider. By limiting transitions to those that remain within valid boundaries, the system eliminates large portions of the state space. This reduction allows the system to focus its processing on a smaller set of viable options, increasing efficiency without sacrificing accuracy. Constraints therefore act as filters that concentrate computational effort where it is most effective.

Sequencing organizes these elements into repeatable pathways. When transitions are applied in a defined order, the system can execute complex transformations through a consistent sequence. This sequence becomes a reusable structure that can be applied to different inputs. The system does not construct a new pathway for each decision. It selects and executes from a set of existing sequences that have been validated within the model.

Leverage also emerges from composability. Smaller structures can be combined to form larger ones, allowing the system to build complex pathways from simpler components. Each component retains its defined behavior, and their combination produces new interactions that are still governed by the same rules. This allows the system to scale its capability without increasing complexity at every level. The structure grows by composition rather than by expansion of individual elements.

Feedback integration strengthens leverage over time. As the system applies its model and observes outcomes, it refines variables, relationships, and constraints. Each refinement improves the accuracy of all pathways that use those components. A single adjustment can therefore affect a wide range of decisions. This creates a compounding effect, where improvements in structure produce improvements across the entire system.

Leverage reduces dependence on brute-force processing. Instead of evaluating large numbers of possibilities through approximation, the system relies on its structured pathways to narrow the search space and guide transformation. This allows it to produce accurate outputs with fewer operations, because the model encodes the relationships that determine how variables interact.

The effect of logic as leverage is most visible under increasing complexity. As the number of variables and interactions grows, unstructured systems require exponentially more effort to maintain alignment. A structured system scales more efficiently because its operations are constrained and reusable. The same logical framework can handle additional complexity without a proportional increase in processing.

Logic does not add capability by itself. It organizes existing capability into a form that can be applied consistently and efficiently. By embedding logic into the architecture of the model, the system converts individual operations into reusable structures. Each execution reinforces these structures, allowing them to be applied across contexts with minimal variation.

A system that uses logic as leverage operates with controlled efficiency. It produces outputs through pathways that have been defined, validated, and refined, reducing the need for reconstruction and minimizing the introduction of error. This allows it to handle a wide range of inputs while maintaining alignment, because the structure that generates its outputs remains stable and reusable across instances.

Logic as a Multiplier

A system multiplies its inputs when the structure that processes those inputs produces effects that extend beyond their initial scale. Logic provides this multiplication by controlling how variables are transformed and how those transformations propagate through the model. The same input, when passed through an unstructured system, produces a limited and inconsistent effect because each step in the pathway introduces variation. When passed through a structured system, that input is expanded through defined relationships, constrained transitions, and preserved sequencing, allowing its influence to extend across multiple variables and states without degradation.

Amplification begins at the point of entry. An input is not treated as an isolated signal. It is mapped into the system's variable structure, where it interacts with existing conditions. The strength of the input is determined not only by its magnitude but by how many relationships it activates. A well-defined model allows a single input to engage multiple pathways simultaneously, producing a coordinated set of changes. Each activated relationship applies a transformation that is consistent with the system's rules, ensuring that the input's effect is extended without distortion.

Propagation carries the input through the model. Each transformation produces a new state that becomes the basis for the next step. Because the relationships are defined and constrained, the propagation remains stable. The system does not lose the signal as it moves through layers of processing. Instead, the signal is translated and extended, influencing additional variables at each stage. This creates a cascade where the initial input produces a sequence of aligned changes rather than a single isolated outcome.

Constraint enforcement ensures that amplification does not become divergence. As the input propagates, each transformation is checked against variable boundaries and relationship conditions. This prevents the system from generating states that fall outside its valid structure. Amplification therefore increases the reach of the input while maintaining alignment with the model. The system expands the effect without allowing it to become unstable.

Composability increases the scale of amplification. Structured pathways can be combined so that the output of one sequence becomes the input to another. This chaining allows the system to extend the influence of a single input across multiple layers of processing. Each layer applies its own transformations, further expanding the effect. The system builds complexity from a small set of inputs by leveraging the interactions between its components.

Selective routing directs amplification toward relevant pathways. Not all relationships should be activated by every input. The system uses conditions to determine which pathways are engaged, focusing processing on areas where the input has the greatest impact. This targeted propagation prevents dilution, ensuring that the amplified effect remains concentrated within the parts of the model that are most affected by the input.

Feedback integration reinforces amplification over time. As the system observes the outcomes produced by its pathways, it refines the relationships that contribute most effectively to desired states. This increases the efficiency of propagation, allowing inputs to produce stronger and more predictable effects. Each refinement improves the system's ability to extend the influence of its inputs without increasing the amount of processing required.

Scaling emerges from repeated application. When the same structured pathways are used across multiple inputs, the system accumulates effects that build on each other. Each input is amplified through the same architecture, and the resulting changes interact within the shared state of the system. This produces compounded outcomes, where the combined effect of multiple inputs exceeds the sum of their individual contributions.

Resource efficiency defines the advantage of multiplication. Instead of increasing input magnitude to achieve larger outcomes, the system increases the effectiveness of its processing. Logic allows the system to extract more impact from the same input by ensuring that each transformation contributes to a coherent progression. This reduces the need for additional inputs while maintaining or increasing the scale of the result.

A system without structured logic cannot sustain amplification. Inputs degrade as they pass through inconsistent transformations, and their effects dissipate across uncoordinated pathways. With logic embedded in its architecture, the system converts each input into a sequence of aligned changes that extend its influence across the model. The result is a multiplication of effect, where the structure of processing determines how far and how effectively an input can propagate.

Identifying Inefficiencies

Inefficiency appears where the system expends resources without producing proportional change in state. It is not defined by effort alone but by the mismatch between transformation and outcome. A pathway consumes time, energy, or attention, yet the resulting state either fails to align with the intended target or requires repeated correction. These mismatches accumulate in the structure as unnecessary transitions, redundant evaluations, and unresolved deviations. Opportunity exists precisely at these points because they represent locations where structural changes can increase output without increasing input.

Detection begins with tracing execution pathways from input to output. The system reconstructs the sequence of transformations applied during a decision and maps how each step altered the state. This trace reveals where progress stalls, where variables are reprocessed without net change, and where transitions produce minimal effect relative to their cost. A step that consistently produces small or reversible changes indicates a weak transformation. It consumes resources but does not move the system meaningfully toward the target state.

Redundancy is a primary source of inefficiency. The system may evaluate the same relationship multiple times under slightly varied representations, or it may maintain parallel pathways that resolve to equivalent outcomes. These duplications arise when variable definitions are not stable or when relationships are not centralized within the structure. Each redundant evaluation increases processing load without expanding capability. Consolidating these pathways into a single, well-defined transformation reduces cost while preserving function.

Latency introduces another form of inefficiency. When there is a delay between action and observable outcome, the system continues to operate without incorporating the effect of its prior execution. This creates overlapping cycles where multiple decisions are made before feedback from earlier ones is integrated. The result is model drift, where the system moves further from alignment because it is operating on outdated state information. Reducing latency, or explicitly accounting for it within the model, restores synchronization between execution and feedback.

Misallocation of resolution also degrades efficiency. The system may apply high-resolution processing to variables that have minimal impact on the final outcome while compressing those that determine critical transitions. This inversion of priority increases computational cost without improving accuracy. Identifying which variables and relationships drive the majority of state change allows the system to concentrate precision where it produces the greatest effect. Lower-impact components can be processed with reduced resolution, freeing resources for critical pathways.

Constraint violations that require downstream correction create hidden inefficiency. When the system allows transitions that fall outside valid boundaries, it must later expend additional effort to correct the resulting state. This introduces extra steps that would not exist if constraints were enforced at the point of transition. Strengthening constraint checks early in the pathway prevents these corrective loops, reducing the total number of operations required to reach a valid state.

Unmodeled variables generate persistent inefficiency. When external factors influence outcomes but are not represented within the model, the system repeatedly encounters deviations it cannot explain. It attempts to compensate through adjustments to existing variables, but these adjustments fail to resolve the underlying cause. The result is a cycle of correction without convergence. Incorporating the missing variables into the structure allows the system to account for their effects directly, eliminating the need for repeated compensation.

Feedback quality determines how quickly inefficiencies are identified. If observations are imprecise or inconsistently mapped to internal variables, the system cannot accurately measure deviation. This obscures the location and magnitude of inefficiencies, delaying correction. Improving measurement and ensuring that observed states align with the model's definitions increases the clarity of the feedback signal, allowing the system to isolate and address inefficiencies more effectively.

Opportunity emerges when inefficiencies are removed or reorganized. Eliminating redundant steps reduces resource consumption. Reordering transitions can shorten pathways, allowing the system to reach target states with fewer operations. Refining variable definitions can simplify relationships, reducing the complexity of each transformation. Each change increases the ratio of output to input, allowing the system to produce greater effect with the same or reduced resources.

A system that continuously identifies inefficiencies converts wasted effort into structured improvement. It does not attempt to increase output by adding more input. It reshapes the pathways that generate output so that each step contributes directly to state change. Over time, this process concentrates effort within the most effective transformations, allowing the system to operate with increasing efficiency while expanding its capability to produce aligned outcomes.

System Design for Output Scaling

A system scales output when its structure allows the same unit of reasoning to produce effects across multiple instances without being rebuilt from scratch each time. This is the difference between linear effort and leverage. In a linear system, every output requires a fresh sequence of attention, analysis, and execution. The pathway is consumed as it is used. In a leveraged system, the pathway is preserved as structure. Once variables are defined, relationships are stabilized, constraints are enforced, and transitions are organized into repeatable sequences, each additional execution draws on the same architecture. Output increases because the system is no longer paying the full construction cost on every pass.

The first requirement is structural persistence. A model must exist independently of the moment in which it is used. If reasoning only occurs as improvised processing in response to immediate inputs, nothing scales. The system may produce acceptable outputs, but each one depends on live effort rather than on reusable structure. To scale, the model must retain its variable definitions, its relationship rules, and its sequencing logic between executions. This allows future inputs to enter an existing architecture rather than forcing the system to reconstruct the pathway each time. What scales is not raw effort. It is the reuse of organized transformations.

Modularity is the next layer. A system cannot scale if every function depends on every other function at the same level of resolution. That creates entanglement, where changing one part forces recalculation of the whole. A scalable system separates its architecture into modules, each responsible for a defined transformation or class of transformations. One module may govern input filtering, another variable construction, another scenario simulation, another output conversion. These modules are connected, but they remain bounded. This boundedness matters because it allows one part of the system to be improved, replaced, or expanded without destabilizing the rest. Scaling requires local modification with global continuity.

Once modules exist, composability becomes the multiplier. A strong system is not built from one large pathway. It is built from smaller structures that can be combined into larger ones. A variable-identification module can feed into a relationship-mapping module. A relationship-mapping module can feed into a simulation module. A simulation module can feed into an execution module. Each module retains its own structure, but when composed, they produce larger pathways that can handle more complex tasks without requiring that complexity to be rebuilt at every layer. This is where leverage begins to compound. The system gains the ability to create increasingly large outputs from a relatively stable set of building blocks.

Constraint architecture is what keeps scaling from becoming collapse. As output increases, the number of reachable states expands. Without strong constraint enforcement, the system begins to generate invalid pathways, incoherent states, and contradictory outputs. Scaling then becomes mere expansion of noise. A leveraged system scales only because its constraints scale with it. Each module enforces boundaries on the variables it manipulates. Each transition preserves continuity. Each composed sequence remains inside the valid state space of the model. This is why constraints are not a drag on output. They are what make higher output possible without losing structural integrity.

Abstraction is another core leverage structure. Once a sequence of operations has been defined and validated, it no longer needs to be processed at full resolution every time. The system can encapsulate it as a higher-order function. This does not mean discarding its internal structure. It means preserving that structure while allowing it to be called as a unit. A five-step reasoning sequence that has been made explicit, tested, and stabilized can later function as a single reusable operation inside a larger model. This is how scale is achieved without overwhelming the system with detail at every level. Abstraction compresses execution while preserving architecture.

Parallelization increases throughput when the system identifies which modules or pathways are independent enough to run simultaneously. Not all transformations require serial execution. Some branches of a model can process distinct inputs or projections at the same time, provided they do not depend on each other's intermediate states. A scalable system maps these dependencies explicitly. It knows where order matters and where it does not. By separating dependent from independent processing, the system increases total output without forcing every pathway through the same bottleneck. The gain is not just speed. It is preservation of resolution while increasing volume.

Feedback scaling is equally important. A system that scales output but cannot scale correction becomes fragile. As more outputs are generated, more deviations appear, and if the system cannot trace those deviations back to the structural components that produced them, error accumulates faster than refinement. A leveraged architecture therefore routes feedback back into modules rather than only into individual instances. If a variable-definition module is flawed, correcting that module improves every pathway that depends on it. If a simulation component is recalibrated, every decision sequence built on that component improves at once. This is one of the deepest forms of leverage: local correction with system-wide effect.

Bottlenecks reveal where leverage is being lost. In any scaling system, certain modules bear more load than others. These modules determine the maximum rate at which outputs can be produced. If a bottleneck remains unresolved, adding more inputs does not increase useful output. It only increases queueing, compression, and distortion around the constrained point. Structural scaling therefore requires continuous bottleneck analysis. The system must identify which transformations consume disproportionate resources, which interfaces create delay, and which modules accumulate unresolved state. Once identified, those bottlenecks can be redesigned, split, abstracted, or parallelized. This is how the architecture preserves increasing returns instead of degrading into congestion.

State management becomes more important as output expands. A system that produces many outputs across multiple modules must maintain a coherent representation of its current state or it loses continuity between executions. Each pathway changes the system, and those changes must be integrated in a way that keeps future decisions aligned with actual conditions. A scalable system therefore does not treat outputs as isolated products. It treats them as transformations of a shared state architecture. That architecture must remain synchronized across modules, across feedback loops, and across time. Without that, scale produces fragmentation instead of leverage.

The real measure of output scaling is not whether the system can do more. It is whether it can do more without proportional increases in reconstruction, correction, and instability. That only happens when structure does the work. Defined variables, reusable modules, composable pathways, constraint-preserving transitions, scalable feedback, and explicit state coordination together form the leverage structures that convert a reasoning system from a sequence of isolated efforts into an architecture capable of persistent multiplication.

Chapter 19

AI and Cognitive Amplification

Cognitive amplification occurs when an external system extends the range, speed, and structural depth of internal reasoning without replacing the underlying model that governs decisions. Artificial intelligence functions as such a system when it is integrated as an extension of the reasoning architecture rather than treated as a source of answers. The distinction is structural. If AI outputs are accepted without passing through the system's variable definitions, relationship constraints, and inference pathways, the result is substitution. If those outputs are processed, reshaped, and validated within the existing model, the result is amplification.

The point of integration begins at representation. The system must translate problems into structured inputs before engaging AI. This involves defining variables, establishing boundaries, and specifying the relationships that need to be evaluated. Without this step, AI receives unstructured input and returns outputs that reflect patterns rather than constrained reasoning. Structured input constrains the output space, allowing the external system to operate within the same architecture that governs internal processing. The quality of amplification is determined by how precisely the system defines this interface.

AI increases throughput by expanding the number of transformations that can be evaluated within a given time frame. It can generate multiple candidate pathways, simulate outcomes across different variable configurations, and explore edge conditions that would be too resource-intensive to process manually. This expansion does not improve the model by itself. It increases the volume of intermediate states that the system can examine. The internal model must still determine which of these states are valid, which relationships hold under constraint, and which pathways remain consistent with the defined structure.

Parallel exploration is one of the primary amplification mechanisms. The system can distribute variations of a problem across multiple AI-generated pathways, each representing a different configuration of variables or assumptions. These pathways are then evaluated against the model's constraints. Invalid pathways are discarded, and valid ones are compared for alignment and efficiency. This process increases the likelihood of identifying optimal or near-optimal solutions without requiring sequential exploration of each possibility.

Compression operates in the opposite direction. AI can reduce complex sequences into more compact representations, allowing the system to store and reuse them as higher-level abstractions. A validated reasoning sequence can be encapsulated and later invoked as a single transformation within a larger pathway. This reduces the cost of re-executing detailed steps while preserving the structure that ensures correctness. Compression therefore converts repeated processing into reusable components, increasing efficiency across the system.

Interface control determines whether amplification remains aligned. The system must enforce its variable definitions and constraints on both input and output. Outputs generated by AI are not directly integrated. They are decomposed into variables, mapped onto the model's structure, and passed through constraint checks. Any element that falls outside defined boundaries is either corrected or discarded. This prevents external outputs from introducing inconsistencies into the system's architecture.

Feedback integration extends to the external system. When AI-generated pathways produce outcomes that align with observed results, the system reinforces the structures that selected those pathways. When they fail, the system adjusts its filtering criteria, input representations, or constraint enforcement. Over time, this creates a calibrated interface where the external system is used in a way that consistently produces usable intermediate states.

Error propagation is a key risk in amplification. Because AI can generate outputs at high volume, any misalignment in the interface or constraint system can produce large numbers of invalid pathways. These errors can overwhelm the system if they are not filtered early. The system must therefore apply constraint checks as close to the point of generation as possible, preventing invalid states from entering deeper levels of processing.

Dependence is another structural risk. If the system begins to rely on AI outputs without maintaining its own model, it loses the ability to validate and refine those outputs. Amplification collapses into substitution, and the system's internal structure degrades. Maintaining an independent model ensures that the external system remains a tool rather than a replacement.

Scaling cognitive output through AI requires alignment between the external system and the internal architecture. The external system increases the range of possible transformations and the speed at which they can be evaluated. The internal system ensures that only valid transformations are integrated into decision pathways. This interaction allows the system to explore more possibilities, process more information, and refine its structure more rapidly than it could alone.

Cognitive amplification is therefore not a function of access to AI. It is a function of how that access is structured. When integrated correctly, AI extends the system's capacity while preserving its integrity. When integrated without structure, it introduces variability that degrades alignment. The system that benefits from amplification is the one that maintains control over its variables, relationships, and constraints while using external processing to expand the space of possible transformations.

AI as Reasoning Extension

A reasoning system retains control when external computation is used to extend its existing structure rather than to substitute for it. Artificial intelligence becomes an extension only when it operates inside the system's defined architecture of variables, relationships, and constraints. The system remains the source of definition and validation. AI becomes a processor that expands transformation capacity. If this boundary is not enforced, the external system begins to supply both structure and output, and the internal model is bypassed. At that point, reasoning is no longer being extended. It is being replaced.

The extension begins at input construction. The system does not pass raw questions or loosely defined problems into AI. It translates them into structured representations, specifying variables, boundaries, and the relationships that need to be evaluated. This translation determines the space in which the external system operates. Without it, the output reflects pattern completion rather than constrained inference. With it, the output is shaped by the same architecture that governs internal reasoning.

AI increases processing capacity by generating candidate transformations. It can expand a single input into multiple pathways, each representing a different sequence of variable interactions or assumptions. These pathways are not decisions. They are intermediate states that require validation. The internal system evaluates each pathway against its constraints, discarding those that violate boundaries and retaining those that remain consistent with the model. This separation preserves control. Generation occurs externally. selection remains internal.

Decomposition is required before integration. Outputs from AI are not accepted as complete units. They are broken down into their component variables and transitions, then mapped onto the system's structure. Each element is checked for alignment with existing definitions. Any mismatch indicates either an invalid pathway or a gap in the model. The system resolves this by either rejecting the output or updating its structure in a controlled way. This prevents external outputs from introducing unverified relationships.

Constraint enforcement defines the boundary of extension. Even when operating at high throughput, the system does not relax its constraints to accommodate external outputs. Variable limits, relationship conditions, and sequence validity are applied uniformly, regardless of source. This ensures that the external system cannot produce states that the internal model would not generate on its own. Extension increases capacity, not the range of acceptable states.

Abstraction allows the system to capture useful external sequences as internal structure. When an AI-generated pathway is validated and produces consistent outcomes, it can be encoded as a reusable component within the model. This converts external computation into internal capability. Over time, the system accumulates these components, reducing its reliance on external generation for similar tasks. The extension therefore contributes to the growth of the internal architecture.

Feedback integration aligns the interface between systems. The internal model tracks which types of structured inputs produce valid external pathways and which do not. It adjusts how it frames problems, how it defines variables, and how it applies constraints to improve the quality of generated transformations. This creates a calibrated interaction where the external system consistently produces outputs that can be integrated with minimal correction.

Error amplification is the primary failure mode. If the system accepts external outputs without decomposition and constraint checking, errors propagate rapidly because of the external system's throughput. Small misalignments in variable definition or relationship logic can produce large volumes of invalid states. These states can overwhelm the internal system, making it difficult to isolate and correct the source of error. Strict interface control prevents this accumulation.

Dependence shifts control away from the system. If the internal model is not maintained and updated independently, the system loses its ability to evaluate external outputs. It begins to rely on the external system for both generation and validation. This removes the structural boundary that defines extension. The system can no longer distinguish between valid and invalid pathways, and its outputs become inconsistent.

A reasoning system that uses AI as an extension maintains its architecture as the primary mechanism of decision-making. External computation increases the number of transformations that can be explored and reduces the time required to evaluate them. The internal model ensures that only those transformations that align with defined variables, relationships, and constraints are incorporated into final outputs. This preserves coherence while expanding capacity.

Extension therefore depends on control. The system must define its inputs, enforce its constraints, and validate its outputs. AI contributes processing power, not authority. When this distinction is maintained, the system gains the ability to operate at greater scale and complexity without losing alignment with its own structure.

Prompting as Structured Thought

A reasoning system receives output in direct proportion to the structure of its input. Prompting is not a peripheral interaction. It is the front end of the reasoning architecture, where variables are defined, boundaries are set, and relationships are specified before any transformation occurs. When input is unstructured, the system expands ambiguity into multiple possible interpretations, each producing different pathways. When input is structured, the system constrains interpretation and forces processing to occur within a defined space. The difference in output is not due to differences in capability. It is due to differences in how the problem is represented at entry.

The construction of a prompt begins with variable definition. Each element of the problem must be expressed as a distinct component with clear boundaries. If variables are merged, implied, or left undefined, the system must infer their structure during processing. This introduces variability, because different inferred structures lead to different outputs. Explicit variables remove this ambiguity. They anchor the reasoning process to a stable representation, ensuring that transformations operate on consistent elements.

Relationship specification follows. Variables do not exist in isolation. The prompt must define how they interact, whether through cause-and-effect chains, constraints, or conditional dependencies. If relationships are omitted, the system fills the gap with pattern-based associations, which may not reflect the intended structure. When relationships are specified, the system processes inputs through defined interactions, producing outputs that align with the intended logic of the model.

Constraint definition limits the solution space. A prompt that does not define constraints allows the system to explore a wide range of possible states, many of which may be irrelevant or invalid. Constraints restrict this space, forcing the system to consider only those pathways that satisfy defined conditions. This increases both efficiency and accuracy, as the system spends fewer resources evaluating pathways that do not meet the requirements.

Sequencing organizes the transformation process. A prompt that specifies the order in which variables should be processed ensures that intermediate states are constructed correctly. Without sequencing, the system may apply transformations in an order that produces inconsistent or incomplete results. By defining the sequence, the prompt controls how the reasoning process unfolds, preserving the integrity of each step.

Resolution determines the depth of processing. A prompt can require high-resolution evaluation of certain variables and relationships while allowing others to be processed at a lower level of detail. This allocation of resolution directs computational resources to the parts of the problem that most influence the outcome. Without this guidance, the system may distribute effort unevenly, reducing efficiency.

Ambiguity introduces branching. When a prompt contains undefined terms, overlapping variables, or unclear relationships, the system generates multiple internal representations to account for the uncertainty. Each representation leads to a different pathway, increasing variability in the output. Reducing ambiguity collapses these branches, allowing the system to follow a single, well-defined pathway.

Feedback from outputs informs prompt refinement. When the system produces results that deviate from expectations, the cause often lies in the structure of the input rather than in the processing itself. Adjusting variable definitions, relationships, or constraints within the prompt changes the pathways that the system can generate. This iterative refinement improves alignment between input and output over time.

Prompting therefore functions as structured thought. It externalizes the internal model into a form that can be processed by the system. The quality of this externalization determines the quality of the resulting output. A well-structured prompt encodes the same architecture that would be used in internal reasoning, allowing the system to extend that reasoning through additional processing capacity.

A system that treats prompting as structured thought maintains control over its outputs. It defines the space in which processing occurs, ensuring that the resulting transformations remain aligned with its model. The output is not a product of the system's capability alone. It is the direct consequence of how the input is constructed, constrained, and sequenced at the point of entry.

Scaling Thought Through Systems

A reasoning system scales when each cycle of processing produces not only an output but an improvement in the structure that generated that output. Thought becomes scalable when it is no longer tied to a single execution instance and instead operates through persistent architecture that can be reused, refined, and extended. Iterative amplification emerges from this process. Each pass through the system modifies variables, strengthens relationships, sharpens constraints, and reorganizes pathways so that subsequent executions produce greater effect with the same or reduced input.

The cycle begins with structured execution. The system applies its current model to transform an input into an output through a defined sequence of variable interactions. This sequence is not discarded after use. It is preserved as a trace, capturing how each transformation contributed to the final state. This trace provides the foundation for amplification because it allows the system to inspect its own behavior at a structural level rather than only observing the outcome.

Comparison follows execution. The system evaluates the difference between the predicted state generated by the model and the observed state produced in reality. This difference is not treated as a general error. It is decomposed into deviations across specific variables and transitions. Each deviation represents a point where the model's representation diverges from the system it is attempting to describe. These points become targets for refinement.

Localization identifies where in the pathway the divergence first occurred. By tracing the sequence of transformations, the system isolates the exact step where predicted and observed states separate. This step may involve an incorrect variable definition, an incomplete relationship, or a constraint that does not reflect actual boundaries. Localization converts a broad mismatch into a specific structural fault that can be addressed directly.

Adjustment modifies the identified component. The system refines the variable, updates the relationship, or corrects the constraint so that the transformation produces a state closer to the observed outcome. This adjustment is applied with precision, leaving other parts of the model unchanged. The goal is to improve alignment without introducing instability elsewhere in the architecture.

Reintegration incorporates the adjustment into the broader system. The updated component is not isolated. It is connected to all pathways that depend on it. This means that a single refinement can influence multiple sequences, improving their accuracy simultaneously. This is where amplification begins to compound. Each correction has system-wide impact because it modifies shared structure rather than a single instance.

Re-execution tests the updated model. The system applies the refined structure to new inputs or repeated conditions, observing whether the deviations decrease. Successful adjustments produce convergence between predicted and observed states. Unsuccessful adjustments generate new deviations, which are then localized and corrected in subsequent cycles. This creates a continuous loop of execution and refinement.

Accumulation across cycles produces amplification. Each iteration improves the model's alignment, allowing it to generate outputs that require fewer corrections. At the same time, the system's pathways become more efficient, as redundant steps are removed and relationships are clarified. The system begins to produce higher-quality outputs at greater speed because its structure has been optimized through repeated refinement.

Scaling occurs because improvements are retained. The system does not relearn the same corrections for each input. It integrates them into its architecture, allowing future executions to benefit from past refinements. This retention converts individual learning events into persistent capability. The system's output capacity increases not by increasing effort but by improving the effectiveness of its structure.

Parallel amplification can occur when multiple pathways are refined simultaneously. Independent components of the model can undergo their own cycles of execution and adjustment, each contributing to the overall improvement of the system. As these components are reintegrated, their combined refinements produce a larger increase in capability than any single pathway could achieve alone.

Constraint stability ensures that amplification remains controlled. As the system evolves, it must maintain the boundaries that define valid states. Adjustments that improve alignment in one area must not violate constraints in another. This requires continuous validation of the model's integrity as it scales, preserving coherence across all pathways.

Iterative amplification transforms thought from a static process into a dynamic system. Each execution contributes to the refinement of the architecture, and each refinement increases the system's ability to produce aligned outputs. Over time, the system becomes more efficient, more accurate, and more capable, not because it processes more information, but because it processes information through an increasingly optimized structure.

Chapter 20

The New Economy of Thinking

The value of thinking shifts when output is no longer limited by individual processing capacity but by the structure that governs how processing occurs. In a system where reasoning can be extended, replicated, and amplified through external computation, the limiting factor is not effort. It is architecture. The economy of thinking reorganizes around the ability to define variables precisely, construct valid relationships, enforce constraints, and design pathways that can be reused and scaled. Those who operate with structured models produce outputs that extend beyond their direct input because their reasoning can be applied repeatedly without reconstruction.

Scarcity moves from information to alignment. Information is abundant and continuously generated, but it does not translate into value without a structure that can filter, organize, and transform it into coherent outputs. A system that lacks structure processes large volumes of input but produces inconsistent results because it cannot maintain stable relationships between variables. A structured system processes less input but extracts more usable signal because each transformation is constrained and aligned. The difference in output is determined by how effectively the system converts information into structured representations.

Leverage becomes the primary driver of output. A system that encodes its reasoning into reusable components can apply the same transformations across multiple inputs. This reduces the marginal cost of each additional output. The initial investment in defining variables, relationships, and constraints produces a persistent architecture that continues to generate value. Each refinement to this architecture improves all future outputs, creating a compounding effect that increases efficiency over time.

Throughput increases with the integration of external processing systems, but this increase only produces value when it is aligned with internal structure. High-volume generation without constraint produces noise. High-volume generation within a defined model produces a range of valid intermediate states that can be evaluated and integrated. The system that can control this interface converts increased throughput into increased capability, while the system that cannot becomes overwhelmed by unstructured output.

Differentiation emerges from model quality. When multiple systems have access to similar information and processing tools, the distinguishing factor is how those tools are used. A system with well-defined variables, accurate relationships, and enforced constraints produces outputs that remain consistent across conditions. A system without these elements produces outputs that vary with context and degrade under complexity. The quality of the model determines the reliability and scalability of the output.

Feedback integration accelerates improvement. As outputs are generated and compared to observed outcomes, the system refines its structure. Each correction improves not only the specific pathway that produced the output but all pathways that share the same components. This creates a compounding effect where improvements propagate across the system, increasing the accuracy and efficiency of future outputs. The rate at which a system can integrate feedback into its architecture determines how quickly it can adapt and improve.

The cost structure of thinking changes as well. In a linear system, each output requires direct effort, and the total cost increases proportionally with the number of outputs. In a leveraged system, the cost is concentrated in building and refining the structure. Once the architecture is established, additional outputs can be generated at a lower marginal cost. This shifts the focus from producing individual outputs to designing systems that can produce outputs consistently and at scale.

Error management becomes more critical as output scales. A system that produces large volumes of output must maintain strict control over its structure to prevent the propagation of error. Small misalignments in variable definitions or relationship logic can produce widespread inconsistencies when applied across many pathways. The system must therefore prioritize accuracy in its core components, ensuring that the foundation of its architecture remains stable as it scales.

Access to tools is no longer a differentiator. The availability of external processing systems means that many systems can generate outputs at high speed. The differentiator is the ability to integrate these tools into a structured model that maintains alignment. Systems that rely on tool output without maintaining internal structure produce inconsistent results. Systems that integrate tools into their architecture produce outputs that are both scalable and reliable.

The economy of thinking therefore rewards structure over effort. Value is created by systems that can define, apply, and refine their models in a way that produces consistent outputs across varying conditions. These systems convert information into structured representations, use those representations to guide processing, and integrate feedback to improve their architecture over time. As a result, they generate outputs that scale in both volume and quality, not because they process more information, but because they process it through a structure that preserves alignment.

Logic as the New Currency

Value shifts when possession of information no longer limits output. In an environment where data is abundant and accessible, holding information does not create advantage. Advantage emerges from the ability to process that information into structured, aligned outputs. Logic becomes the currency because it determines how effectively a system can convert raw input into usable transformation. The system that can define variables, enforce relationships, and constrain outcomes produces results that extend beyond what it holds. The system that cannot remains dependent on the volume of what it possesses.

Processing defines how inputs are transformed. A system receives information, but the form in which that information is represented determines what can be done with it. If inputs are unstructured, they remain static. They cannot be reliably combined, compared, or extended. When inputs are translated into defined variables with clear boundaries, they become components that can be manipulated within the model. This translation is the first step in converting possession into function. Without it, information accumulates but does not integrate.

Relationships determine how value is extracted. Information does not produce output in isolation. It produces output when it is connected through defined interactions. A system that encodes how variables influence each other can generate new states from existing inputs. This allows it to extend beyond what it directly holds. The same set of inputs can produce different outputs depending on how relationships are structured. This is where processing overtakes possession. The structure of interaction matters more than the volume of stored data.

Constraint enforcement defines validity. In a system without constraints, any combination of variables can be produced, but most of those combinations will not correspond to real or usable states. Constraints limit the system to transformations that remain within defined boundaries. This allows the system to filter outputs, ensuring that what it produces maintains coherence with the model. Possession cannot provide this filtering. Only structured processing can determine which outputs are valid.

Sequencing converts structure into action. Defined variables and relationships must be applied in a controlled order to produce consistent outcomes. The sequence determines how intermediate states are constructed and how transformations accumulate. A system with strong sequencing can reproduce its outputs across different inputs because the pathway remains stable. This repeatability is a form of stored value. It allows the system to generate outputs without reconstructing the process each time.

Leverage emerges when processing is reusable. Once a system has defined its variables, relationships, constraints, and sequences, it can apply them across multiple inputs. Each new input does not require a new model. It passes through the existing architecture, producing outputs that reflect the same structured reasoning. This reduces the marginal cost of each additional output. Possession scales linearly. Processing scales through reuse.

Feedback integration compounds value. When outputs are compared to observed outcomes, the system refines its structure. Each refinement improves the way variables are defined, how relationships are applied, and how constraints are enforced. These improvements affect all future processing. A single correction can increase the quality of many outputs. This creates a compounding effect where the system's value grows over time through refinement of its processing architecture.

Throughput amplifies this effect when aligned with structure. A system that can process more inputs per unit time increases its output, but only if those inputs are handled within a defined model. High throughput without structure produces volume without coherence. High throughput with structure produces a large number of valid transformations that can be integrated into the system's state. The combination of processing capacity and structured logic determines how much value can be generated from available information.

Possession remains static. Information can be stored, retrieved, and referenced, but without structured processing, it does not produce aligned outputs. Processing converts static information into dynamic capability. It allows the system to generate new states, adapt to changing conditions, and refine its own structure over time. This is why logic functions as currency. It governs the transformation of input into output, and therefore determines how much value can be extracted from the same underlying information.

A system that prioritizes processing over possession invests in its architecture. It develops the ability to define, connect, and constrain variables in a way that produces consistent results. As this architecture improves, the system's outputs scale in both quantity and quality, independent of the amount of information it holds. Value is no longer tied to accumulation. It is tied to the structure that determines how that accumulation is used.

Value Creation Through Structure

Information does not produce value in its raw state. It exists as unbounded signal, fragmented across contexts, formats, and levels of resolution. Value emerges only when that information is organized into a structure that allows it to be transformed, combined, and applied. The act of organizing information is not categorization for convenience. It is the construction of a system in which variables are defined, relationships are stabilized, and constraints are enforced so that information can participate in coherent transformations. Without this structure, information accumulates but does not integrate, and the system remains incapable of producing consistent outputs.

The process begins with variable extraction. Information is decomposed into discrete elements that can be defined with clear boundaries. Each variable must represent a stable unit that can be referenced consistently across contexts. If boundaries are unclear, the same piece of information may be interpreted differently in different parts of the system, creating inconsistency. By defining variables precisely, the system creates a set of components that can be manipulated without ambiguity. This transforms raw information into usable parts.

Relationship mapping connects these variables into a functional network. Information gains value when it can influence other information through defined interactions. These interactions must be explicit. The system specifies how a change in one variable alters the state of another, under what conditions that interaction occurs, and what form the resulting transformation takes. When relationships are left implicit, the system relies on pattern recognition to fill the gaps, which introduces variability. Explicit mapping stabilizes these interactions, allowing the system to generate predictable outcomes.

Constraint definition limits the system to valid states. Not all combinations of variables and relationships produce meaningful or usable results. Constraints define the boundaries within which transformations are allowed to occur. These boundaries ensure that the system does not generate states that violate its internal logic or external reality. By enforcing constraints, the system reduces the space of possible outputs to those that maintain coherence, increasing the density of useful information within its processing.

Sequencing organizes how transformations unfold. Variables and relationships must be applied in a specific order to produce consistent results. The system defines this order, ensuring that each transformation builds on a valid intermediate state. Without sequencing, operations may occur in an order that produces incomplete or contradictory outcomes. Structured sequencing converts a set of relationships into a pathway that can be executed repeatedly with consistent results.

Abstraction compresses complexity. Once a sequence of transformations has been defined and validated, it can be represented as a higher-level unit within the system. This allows the system to reuse complex operations without reprocessing each internal step. Abstraction reduces the cognitive and computational load required to generate outputs, while preserving the underlying structure that ensures correctness. This enables the system to scale its processing without losing control over its architecture.

Integration allows organized information to function across contexts. Variables and relationships defined in one part of the system must be compatible with those in other parts. This requires a shared representation of state, where all components operate on consistent definitions. Integration ensures that outputs from one pathway can serve as inputs to another, allowing the system to build larger transformations from smaller ones. Without integration, information remains isolated within local structures, limiting its utility.

Feedback refines the organization over time. As the system generates outputs and compares them to observed outcomes, it identifies where its structure does not align with reality. These discrepancies are traced back to variable definitions, relationship mappings, or constraint boundaries. Adjustments are made at these points, improving the system's ability to organize information in a way that produces accurate transformations. Each refinement increases the value that can be extracted from the same underlying information.

Redundancy reduction increases efficiency. When information is organized poorly, the system may represent the same concept in multiple ways or process the same relationship repeatedly. This increases resource consumption without improving output. By consolidating variables and centralizing relationships, the system reduces duplication, allowing each piece of information to contribute more effectively to the overall process.

Value creation through structure is therefore a function of how information is organized into a system that can act on it. The system converts raw data into defined variables, connects those variables through explicit relationships, limits transformations through constraints, and sequences operations into repeatable pathways. This organization allows information to be used rather than stored, producing outputs that reflect the structure of the system rather than the volume of its inputs.

A system that organizes information effectively does not require more data to produce better results. It extracts more value from the data it already has by structuring it in a way that supports transformation. Over time, as this structure is refined and expanded, the system's ability to generate aligned outputs increases, demonstrating that value is not inherent in information itself but in the architecture that determines how that information is used.

Market Advantage Through Reasoning

A system differentiates when it produces outputs that remain aligned under conditions where other systems degrade. In an environment where access to information and tools is widely distributed, advantage does not come from what is available. It comes from how consistently and accurately a system can transform inputs into outcomes. Reasoning defines this transformation. The system that maintains stable variables, enforces relationships, and preserves constraints under changing conditions produces outputs that can be relied on. This reliability is the basis of differentiation because it reduces variance where others introduce it.

Differentiation begins with model integrity. A system that operates from clearly defined variables and explicit relationships maintains continuity between inputs and outputs. When conditions shift, the model adapts through adjustment of its structure rather than through ad hoc responses. This preserves coherence across decisions. A system without this integrity relies on pattern matching or heuristic shortcuts, which produce acceptable outputs under familiar conditions but break under variation. The difference is not visible in stable environments. It appears when the system is forced outside its default patterns.

Consistency across scale amplifies this effect. As the volume of decisions increases, small structural differences in reasoning produce large differences in aggregate output. A system that applies the same defined pathways across instances maintains alignment as it scales. Each additional decision reinforces the structure rather than introducing variation. A system that reconstructs its reasoning for each instance accumulates inconsistency. Over time, these inconsistencies compound, creating divergence between expected and actual outcomes.

Signal extraction is another point of differentiation. Information environments contain both relevant and irrelevant inputs. A structured system filters inputs through its variable definitions and constraints, isolating the elements that affect the outcome. This reduces noise and concentrates processing on signals that drive state change. An unstructured system processes a broader range of inputs without clear filtering, diluting the effect of relevant information and increasing the likelihood of incorrect transformations.

Response time under complexity reveals structural strength. As the number of variables and interactions increases, systems that rely on unstructured processing experience exponential growth in required effort. They slow down or simplify their reasoning, reducing accuracy. A structured system manages complexity through modular pathways, composable components, and constraint enforcement. It maintains both speed and accuracy because its architecture limits the number of valid transformations that must be considered.

Feedback utilization determines how quickly differentiation increases. A system that integrates feedback into its structure improves with each cycle of execution. Errors are localized, adjustments are applied, and the updated components influence all future decisions. This creates a compounding effect where the system's performance improves faster than systems that treat feedback as isolated correction. Over time, the gap widens because one system accumulates structural improvements while the other repeats the same errors.

Adaptability without loss of coherence is critical. Differentiation is not achieved by rigid adherence to a fixed model. It is achieved by maintaining structure while allowing controlled modification of that structure in response to new conditions. The system updates variable definitions, relationship mappings, and constraints while preserving the integrity of its pathways. This allows it to operate effectively in changing environments without introducing instability.

Error containment further separates systems. In a structured model, errors are localized to specific components and can be corrected without affecting the entire system. In an unstructured model, errors propagate because there is no clear boundary between components. This leads to widespread degradation when a single assumption fails. Containment allows the system to maintain performance even when parts of the model require adjustment.

Differentiation ultimately reflects how a system manages transformation. It is not determined by the amount of information processed or the speed at which outputs are generated. It is determined by the alignment between the system's internal structure and the external conditions it operates within. A system that preserves this alignment produces outputs that remain consistent, scalable, and adaptable.

Market advantage emerges from this consistency. When outputs can be predicted, reproduced, and improved through structured reasoning, the system becomes reliable under a wide range of conditions. This reliability reduces risk, increases efficiency, and allows the system to operate at scale without degradation. In environments where many systems have access to the same inputs, the one that can transform those inputs through a stable and adaptable structure establishes differentiation through its ability to maintain alignment where others cannot.

PART VII

THE COGNITIVE DIVIDE

Chapter 21

Thinkers vs Non-Thinkers

The distinction between thinkers and non-thinkers is structural, not intellectual. It is defined by how a system processes inputs, not by how much information it holds or how quickly it produces outputs. A thinker operates through a defined architecture of variables, relationships, constraints, and sequences. A non-thinker operates through pattern recognition, association, and reaction. Both systems can produce outputs that appear similar under simple conditions, but they diverge as complexity increases because one is grounded in structure and the other is driven by approximation.

A thinker begins with representation. Inputs are translated into defined variables with clear boundaries. This allows the system to operate on stable components that can be manipulated consistently across contexts. A non-thinker does not perform this translation. Inputs remain in their original form, often blended with prior patterns and associations. This creates ambiguity at the point of entry, where multiple interpretations of the same input can exist simultaneously. The system proceeds without resolving this ambiguity, leading to variability in output.

Relationship handling separates the two further. A thinker encodes how variables interact, specifying conditions under which one variable influences another. These relationships are applied consistently, producing outputs that reflect the structure of the model. A non-thinker relies on learned associations between inputs and outputs. These associations may approximate relationships but are not explicitly defined.

As a result, they fail when conditions differ from those under which the associations were formed.

Constraint enforcement defines validity. A thinker limits transformations to those that remain within defined boundaries. This ensures that outputs correspond to states that are consistent with the model. A non-thinker does not enforce constraints explicitly. It may generate outputs that appear plausible but fall outside valid boundaries because there is no mechanism to filter them. This leads to outputs that are internally coherent but externally misaligned.

Sequencing organizes processing. A thinker applies transformations in a defined order, ensuring that each step builds on a valid intermediate state. This preserves continuity and allows the system to trace how an output was generated. A non-thinker processes inputs through loosely ordered associations, where the sequence of transformations is not explicitly controlled. This makes it difficult to trace the origin of an output or to identify where an error occurred.

Feedback integration determines improvement. A thinker uses deviations between predicted and observed outcomes to refine its structure. Errors are localized to specific variables, relationships, or constraints and corrected in a way that improves all future outputs. A non-thinker may recognize that an output was incorrect but lacks the structure to identify why. Corrections are applied at the surface level, often through adjustment of associations, which does not address the underlying cause of error.

Scalability reveals the long-term difference. As the number of variables and interactions increases, a thinker maintains alignment because its structure limits the number of valid pathways. A non-thinker experiences exponential growth in possible associations, leading to increased variability and reduced reliability. The system compensates by simplifying inputs or relying on heuristics, which further reduces accuracy.

Adaptability also differs in form. A thinker modifies its structure in response to new information, updating variable definitions, relationships, and constraints while preserving overall coherence. A non-thinker adapts by forming new associations, which may conflict with existing ones. This creates internal inconsistency, where different parts of the system produce outputs that do not align with each other.

Error containment is a direct consequence of structure. In a thinker, errors are localized and corrected without affecting unrelated parts of the model. In a non-thinker, errors propagate because there are no clear boundaries between components. A single incorrect association can influence multiple outputs, creating widespread inconsistency.

The difference is most visible under conditions that require precision, consistency, and scalability. A thinker produces outputs that remain aligned across varying inputs because its structure governs how transformations occur. A non-thinker produces outputs that vary with context because its processing is driven by patterns rather than defined relationships.

This distinction is not fixed. A system can move from non-thinking to thinking by developing structure. It can define variables, map relationships, enforce constraints, and organize sequences. As this structure is built and refined, the system's outputs become more consistent and scalable. The transition is not a change in intelligence. It is a change in architecture.

A system that operates as a thinker maintains control over its processing. It generates outputs through pathways that can be traced, validated, and improved. This allows it to operate effectively under increasing complexity, producing results that reflect its structure rather than the variability of its inputs.

Structured vs Unstructured Systems

Divergence between systems emerges from how they organize transformation, not from differences in input or intent. Two systems can receive the same information and produce outputs that appear similar under simple conditions, yet separate rapidly as complexity increases. The difference is encoded in structure. A structured system defines variables, stabilizes relationships, enforces constraints, and sequences transformations in a controlled manner. An unstructured system processes inputs through loosely connected associations, where variables are implied, relationships are inferred, and constraints are inconsistently applied. This difference determines how each system behaves as conditions change.

A structured system begins with stable representation. Inputs are decomposed into variables with clear boundaries that remain consistent across contexts. These variables act as fixed reference points, allowing transformations to be applied without reinterpretation. An unstructured system does not maintain this stability. Variables shift depending on context, overlap with each other, or remain undefined. As a result, each new input can alter the internal representation, forcing the system to reconstruct its processing pathway. This instability at the level of representation is the first source of divergence.

Relationship handling amplifies the separation. In a structured system, interactions between variables are explicitly defined and applied under known conditions. This creates predictable propagation of change, where the effect of a transformation can be traced through the model. In an unstructured system, relationships are implicit and often derived from pattern similarity. These relationships may approximate correct interactions in familiar scenarios but fail when conditions differ. The system cannot reliably predict how changes will propagate, leading to outputs that vary across similar inputs.

Constraint enforcement determines the validity of generated states. A structured system limits transformations to those that remain within defined boundaries, preventing the creation of states that violate its internal logic or external conditions. An unstructured system lacks consistent constraint application, allowing transformations that appear coherent but fall outside valid ranges. These invalid states may not be immediately obvious, but they accumulate and interact, increasing divergence over time.

Sequencing organizes how transformations unfold. In a structured system, operations occur in a defined order, ensuring that each step builds on a valid intermediate state. This preserves continuity and allows the system to trace its reasoning. An unstructured system applies transformations in a loosely ordered manner, where the sequence is influenced by association rather than by defined pathways. This creates discontinuities, where intermediate states do not align with the requirements of subsequent steps, producing inconsistent outputs.

Feedback integration controls the rate of divergence. A structured system compares predicted and observed outcomes, localizes deviations, and adjusts its variables, relationships, or constraints accordingly. These adjustments improve all pathways that depend on the modified components, reducing future divergence. An unstructured system may detect that an output is incorrect but lacks the structure to identify the source of error. Corrections are applied at the surface level, often by altering associations, which does not address the underlying cause. Divergence therefore persists and compounds.

Scaling exposes the full extent of separation. As the number of variables and interactions increases, a structured system maintains alignment because its constraints limit the number of valid pathways. The system processes complexity through organized components, preserving both accuracy and efficiency. An unstructured system experiences a rapid increase in possible associations, leading to a combinatorial expansion of pathways. Without constraints, the system cannot manage this expansion, resulting in increased variability and reduced reliability.

Error propagation differs fundamentally between the two. In a structured system, errors are localized to specific components and can be corrected without affecting unrelated pathways. In an unstructured system, errors spread because there are no clear boundaries between components. A single incorrect assumption can influence multiple outputs, creating widespread inconsistency. This propagation accelerates divergence as the system continues to operate.

Temporal accumulation reinforces the separation. Each execution in a structured system refines the model, reducing future error and increasing alignment. Each execution in an unstructured system may introduce new inconsistencies, which interact with existing ones. Over time, the structured system converges toward stable performance, while the unstructured system drifts further from alignment.

Divergence is therefore not an abrupt event. It is the cumulative result of how a system processes information at every step. A structured system maintains coherence because its architecture governs transformation. An unstructured system loses coherence because its processing lacks defined boundaries and consistent relationships. As conditions become more complex and the number of interactions increases, the gap between the two systems widens, revealing the underlying difference in how they organize and execute reasoning.

Adaptability and Model Updating

Adaptability is determined by whether a system can modify its internal structure in response to changing conditions while preserving coherence across its operations. A dynamic system updates variables, relationships, and constraints as new information alters the state space it operates within. A static system preserves its existing structure regardless of input, forcing new conditions to be interpreted through outdated representations. Both systems can produce outputs, but only one maintains alignment as the environment shifts. The difference is not in the amount of information processed. It is in whether the model itself is allowed to change.

A dynamic system treats its model as a working structure rather than a fixed reference. Each execution produces not only an output but a comparison between predicted and observed states. Deviations are decomposed into specific variables and transitions, allowing the system to identify where its representation no longer matches reality. These discrepancies trigger targeted updates. Variable definitions may be refined to reflect new boundaries, relationships may be adjusted to capture previously unmodeled interactions, and constraints may be tightened or expanded to match observed limits. The model evolves through these localized modifications, maintaining continuity while increasing accuracy.

A static system does not perform this structural update. It processes new inputs through existing variables and relationships, even when those elements no longer reflect the current environment. Deviations between predicted and observed outcomes are either ignored or explained through surface-level adjustments, such as reinterpreting inputs or modifying outputs without altering the underlying model. This preserves short-term consistency but introduces long-term misalignment, as the system continues to operate on representations that no longer correspond to the system it is attempting to model.

Feedback integration is the mechanism that enables dynamic updating. The system must capture outcomes, translate them into its internal variable structure, and compare them against predictions. This comparison produces a signal that indicates where the model diverges from observed behavior. The system then traces this signal back through its pathways to localize the source of error. Without this traceability, updates cannot be applied precisely, and the system risks altering unrelated components, introducing instability.

Temporal sensitivity influences how updates are applied. A dynamic system distinguishes between transient fluctuations and persistent changes. It requires consistency across multiple observations before making significant modifications, preventing overreaction to noise. At the same time, it maintains the ability to respond quickly when deviations are consistent and large, ensuring that the model does not lag behind the environment. This balance allows the system to remain both stable and responsive.

Constraint management ensures that updates do not destabilize the system. When variables or relationships are modified, the system must verify that these changes remain consistent with existing constraints. If a modification introduces a violation, the system either adjusts the change or redefines the constraint in a controlled manner. This preserves the integrity of the model as it evolves, preventing the accumulation of conflicting elements.

Propagation extends the effect of updates across the system. When a component is modified, all pathways that depend on that component are influenced. This allows a single adjustment to improve multiple sequences, increasing the efficiency of the updating process. The system leverages this propagation to refine its architecture without requiring separate corrections for each pathway.

A static system lacks this propagation because it does not update its structure. Each new input is processed independently, and any adjustments made are not integrated into a persistent model. This prevents the system from accumulating improvements over time. It may produce acceptable outputs in isolated cases, but it does not increase its capability across executions.

Adaptability becomes critical as conditions change. A dynamic system maintains alignment by continuously updating its model to reflect new states and interactions. It preserves the connection between its internal structure and the external environment. A static system loses this connection over time, as its fixed model becomes increasingly misaligned with the conditions it operates within.

Dynamic cognition therefore treats reasoning as an evolving process. The system's structure is not static. It is continuously refined through feedback, ensuring that its variables, relationships, and constraints remain accurate representations of the environment. Static cognition treats reasoning as a fixed process, applying the same structure regardless of change. The result is divergence between the model and reality.

A system that maintains dynamic updating retains its ability to produce aligned outputs across varying conditions. It does not rely on initial correctness. It relies on continuous correction. Each execution contributes to the refinement of the model, allowing the system to adapt without losing coherence. This is the basis of sustained performance in environments where change is constant and unavoidable.

Opportunity Recognition

Opportunity appears where the underlying structure of a system is misread, ignored, or only partially represented. Most systems operate on surface patterns, reacting to visible signals without resolving the variables and relationships that generate those signals. This creates gaps between how a system behaves and how it is perceived. A structured system identifies these gaps by reconstructing the architecture beneath the surface, mapping how inputs propagate through variables, constraints, and interactions to produce outcomes. Where this internal structure differs from the dominant interpretation, opportunity exists.

Recognition begins with representation. Inputs that appear as undifferentiated information are decomposed into variables with clear boundaries. This process reveals components that are otherwise blended together, allowing the system to isolate what is actually changing and what remains constant. When others treat a signal as a single unit, the structured system separates it into parts, exposing internal variation that can be acted on. This separation is the first step in identifying misalignment between perception and mechanism.

Relationship mapping exposes hidden interactions. Surface analysis often assumes direct, linear connections between inputs and outcomes. In reality, most systems operate through multi-step pathways where intermediate variables mediate the effect. By defining these pathways explicitly, the system identifies points where influence is concentrated or where small changes produce disproportionate effects. These points represent leverage, where intervention can alter outcomes more efficiently than acting on the surface variable.

Constraint analysis further refines recognition. Every system operates within boundaries that limit possible states. These constraints are often implicit and therefore overlooked. By identifying them, the system reduces the range of valid transformations and focuses on the subset of states that can actually occur. This reveals where expectations diverge from reality, as many perceived possibilities fall outside the constrained space. Opportunity emerges where others allocate resources toward states that cannot be reached or fail to recognize states that are permitted but unexploited.

Temporal sequencing reveals delayed effects. In many systems, the relationship between action and outcome is separated by time, creating a disconnect between cause and observed result. Systems that operate on immediate feedback fail to connect these delayed interactions, leading to incorrect conclusions about what drives change. By mapping sequences across time, the structured system links actions to outcomes that occur later, identifying causal pathways that are not visible in short-term analysis. This allows it to act on early-stage variables before their effects become widely recognized.

Error patterns provide another signal. When a system consistently produces outcomes that deviate from expectations, the source of error often lies in an incorrect model of its structure. By analyzing where these deviations occur, the system identifies which variables or relationships are being misrepresented. These misrepresentations indicate areas where prevailing models are incomplete or incorrect. Correcting them reveals pathways that others are not using, creating opportunity.

Information asymmetry is not always about access. It is often about interpretation. Multiple systems may have access to the same data, but only those that can organize it into a coherent structure can extract its full value. The difference lies in how variables are defined, how relationships are mapped, and how constraints are enforced. A system that performs these steps gains an advantage not by possessing more information, but by using the same information more effectively.

Execution converts recognition into outcome. Identifying structure is necessary but not sufficient. The system must apply its model to generate actions that exploit the identified gaps. These actions are based on the same structured pathways used for recognition, ensuring that execution remains aligned with the model. As the system acts, it generates feedback that further refines its understanding, reinforcing its ability to identify similar opportunities in the future.

Opportunity recognition therefore depends on structural perception. It requires the system to move beyond surface patterns and reconstruct the mechanisms that produce them. By defining variables, mapping relationships, enforcing constraints, and sequencing interactions, the system reveals discrepancies between appearance and function. These discrepancies are where opportunity resides, because they represent points where the system can act in ways that others do not, producing outcomes that are not accessible through unstructured processing.

Chapter 22

Compounding Advantage

Compounding advantage emerges when improvements to a system's structure persist and propagate across future executions, increasing output without requiring proportional increases in input. The system does not rely on isolated gains. It accumulates structural refinements that alter how all subsequent transformations occur. Each adjustment to variables, relationships, constraints, or sequencing affects not only the immediate pathway but every pathway that depends on those components. Over time, these refinements interact, producing a rate of improvement that exceeds linear accumulation.

The process begins with retention. A system must preserve the changes it makes to its structure. If refinements are applied only at the level of individual execution and are not integrated into the model, they do not compound. They remain isolated corrections that must be repeated. A compounding system incorporates each validated adjustment into its architecture, ensuring that future executions begin from an improved state. This retention converts temporary improvement into persistent capability.

Propagation extends the effect of each refinement. When a variable definition is clarified, every relationship that uses that variable becomes more precise. When a relationship is corrected, every sequence that includes that interaction produces more accurate intermediate states. When a constraint is refined, the entire state space is adjusted, eliminating invalid pathways across the system. This interconnected structure allows a single change to influence multiple components, multiplying its impact.

Consistency across execution is required for compounding to take hold. The system must apply the same structured pathways repeatedly so that refinements can accumulate within them. If the system reconstructs its reasoning for each instance, there is no stable structure in which improvements can be embedded. Consistency ensures that the same components are used across executions, allowing changes to those components to affect future outputs.

Feedback integration drives the accumulation of advantage. Each execution produces a comparison between predicted and observed states. Deviations are localized to specific components and corrected. These corrections are then integrated into the model, improving its alignment. The system repeats this cycle, using each deviation as input for refinement. Over time, the frequency and magnitude of deviations decrease, and the system's outputs converge toward consistent alignment with the environment.

Efficiency gains emerge as redundant or ineffective transformations are removed. As the system refines its structure, it identifies pathways that do not contribute meaningfully to state change or that introduce unnecessary complexity. These pathways are simplified or eliminated, reducing the number of operations required to produce an output. The system becomes faster and more efficient, not by increasing processing capacity, but by improving the organization of its transformations.

Error reduction compounds alongside efficiency. Early refinements address the most significant sources of deviation, producing large improvements in output quality. Subsequent refinements target smaller discrepancies, further increasing precision. Because each refinement builds on previous ones, the system's error rate decreases at an accelerating pace. This creates a widening gap between the system and those that do not integrate feedback into their structure.

Scalability amplifies compounding advantage. As the system processes more inputs, it generates more opportunities for refinement. Each additional execution contributes data that can be used to improve the model. Because refinements are integrated into the structure, the benefits of each improvement are applied across all future outputs. This creates a feedback loop where increased scale leads to increased refinement, which in turn improves the system's ability to handle additional scale.

Constraint stability ensures that compounding remains controlled. As the system evolves, it must maintain the boundaries that define valid states. Refinements that improve alignment in one area must not introduce violations in another. The system continuously verifies that its structure remains coherent, preserving the integrity of its pathways as it accumulates changes.

Temporal accumulation defines the long-term effect. A system that consistently integrates refinements into its structure increases its capability over time, even if each individual improvement is small. These incremental changes interact, producing a level of performance that would not be achievable through isolated adjustments. The advantage compounds because each improvement alters the starting point for the next execution.

A system that achieves compounding advantage operates from an architecture that improves itself through use. It does not rely on external increases in input to produce better outputs. It relies on the continuous refinement of its structure, where each execution contributes to a more accurate, efficient, and scalable model. Over time, this process produces a system that generates outputs with increasing reliability and effectiveness, reflecting the accumulated impact of its structural improvements.

Accumulation of Better Decisions

A system diverges over time based on how consistently its decisions remain aligned with the structure that governs valid outcomes. Each decision is not an isolated event. It modifies the system's state, alters the conditions for subsequent decisions, and either reinforces or degrades the pathways that will be used again. When decisions are produced through structured reasoning, they move the system into states that preserve alignment with its variables, relationships, and constraints.

When decisions are produced through approximation or inconsistency, they introduce small deviations that shift the system away from valid states. These deviations accumulate, producing divergence that becomes visible only after multiple iterations.

The process begins with state transition. Each decision moves the system from one state to another through a defined sequence of transformations. The quality of that transition determines whether the new state remains within the valid space defined by the model. A well-aligned decision produces a state that supports future decisions, maintaining consistency in variable definitions and relationships. A misaligned decision produces a state that contains internal inconsistencies, which must either be corrected or carried forward into subsequent processing.

Compounding emerges from dependency. Each new decision operates on the state produced by prior decisions. If the system remains aligned, each step reinforces the structure, allowing subsequent decisions to be made with greater accuracy and less correction. If the system drifts, each new decision is made from a degraded starting point, increasing the likelihood of further misalignment. The effect is multiplicative rather than additive. Small differences in early decisions produce large differences in later states because each step builds on the previous one.

Error accumulation follows from unresolved deviation. When a system fails to localize and correct errors at the point where they occur, those errors become embedded in the state. Subsequent decisions must operate within this altered structure, often compensating for inconsistencies rather than resolving them. This introduces additional transformations that would not exist in an aligned system, increasing complexity and reducing efficiency. Over time, the system becomes dominated by corrective pathways rather than productive ones.

Path dependence reinforces divergence. Once a system enters a particular state trajectory, the set of available future states is constrained by that trajectory. Decisions that might have been possible from an earlier state may no longer be reachable. This limits the system's ability to recover from misalignment without significant restructuring. A system that consistently produces aligned decisions maintains access to a broader set of valid states, preserving flexibility.

Signal degradation affects perception of divergence. As the system moves further from alignment, its ability to detect deviation decreases because its internal model no longer accurately represents the environment. This creates a feedback loop where misaligned decisions appear acceptable within the system's current representation, allowing divergence to continue unchecked. A structured system maintains accurate mapping between internal variables and external conditions, preserving its ability to detect and correct deviation.

Efficiency differences widen over time. A system that accumulates aligned decisions reduces the need for corrective transformations, allowing more resources to be directed toward productive pathways. A system that accumulates misaligned decisions increases its reliance on correction, consuming resources without advancing toward target states. The gap in efficiency becomes a direct result of the accumulated quality of decisions.

Recovery cost increases with divergence. Early deviations can be corrected with small adjustments to variables or relationships. As divergence grows, correction requires larger structural changes, including redefinition of variables, reorganization of relationships, and re-sequencing of pathways. These changes are more complex and disruptive, making recovery more difficult. A system that maintains alignment avoids these large corrections by addressing deviations as they occur.

Temporal scale reveals the full effect. In short sequences, differences between aligned and misaligned decisions may appear minimal. Over extended sequences, the compounding nature of state transitions produces distinct trajectories. One system converges toward stable, efficient, and predictable outcomes. The other drifts into increasing inconsistency, requiring more effort to maintain function.

The accumulation of better decisions is therefore a structural process. It depends on the system's ability to produce aligned transitions, integrate feedback, and correct deviations at their source. Each decision contributes to the system's trajectory, shaping the conditions under which future decisions are made. Over time, this produces divergence between systems, not because of isolated differences, but because of the cumulative effect of how each system processes and applies its decisions.

Cognitive Compounding

Cognitive compounding occurs when incremental improvements to a system's reasoning structure persist and influence all future processing. The magnitude of each improvement is often small at the point of change. Its effect becomes large because it is applied repeatedly across subsequent executions. The system does not rely on singular breakthroughs. It accumulates adjustments to variables, relationships, constraints, and sequencing, allowing each refinement to modify how every future decision is constructed. Scale emerges from repetition of improved structure, not from increases in input.

The mechanism begins with local correction. A deviation between predicted and observed outcomes is traced to a specific component of the model. The system refines that component so that the same transformation produces a state closer to observed reality. This correction is narrow in scope. It targets one variable definition, one relationship condition, or one constraint boundary. The immediate effect is limited to the pathway where the deviation occurred. The compounding effect appears when that component is reused.

Reuse distributes the improvement. The corrected component exists within multiple pathways that share the same structure. When the system executes those pathways again, each one incorporates the refined behavior. A single adjustment therefore modifies multiple sequences without requiring separate intervention. This distribution is what allows small changes to scale. The improvement is not applied once. It is embedded into the architecture and executed repeatedly.

Iteration amplifies the effect. Each execution cycle produces additional feedback, revealing smaller discrepancies that were not visible before. The system applies further refinements, each one reducing residual error. These refinements interact. Earlier corrections create conditions where later corrections become more effective, because the system's representation is closer to the actual structure it is modeling. The result is a sequence of improvements that build on each other rather than operating independently.

Error reduction compounds alongside accuracy. As the system refines its components, the frequency of large deviations decreases. Remaining errors are smaller and more localized, making them easier to identify and correct. This reduces the cost of future refinement cycles, allowing the system to allocate more resources to productive transformations rather than corrective ones. Over time, the system transitions from correcting major misalignments to optimizing fine-grained behavior.

Efficiency gains follow structural clarity. When variables are precisely defined and relationships are correctly mapped, unnecessary transformations are removed. The system no longer processes redundant pathways or compensates for inconsistencies. Each step contributes directly to state change, reducing the total number of operations required to produce an output. These efficiency gains are not isolated. They apply across all pathways that use the refined components, increasing throughput without additional input.

Propagation ensures that improvements are not lost. Each refinement is integrated into the model rather than applied at the surface level. This integration means that future executions begin from an improved baseline. The system does not need to rediscover the same correction. It operates with the updated structure as its default state. This persistence is what allows improvements to accumulate rather than reset.

Temporal accumulation defines the scaling effect. Over a small number of iterations, the impact of individual refinements may appear limited. Over extended sequences, the repeated application of these refinements produces a substantial increase in performance. The system's outputs become more accurate, more consistent, and more efficient, not because any single change was large, but because many small changes have been applied across many executions.

Constraint stability maintains control during compounding. As the system evolves, it must ensure that refinements do not introduce inconsistencies in other parts of the model. Each adjustment is validated against existing constraints, preserving coherence across the architecture. This prevents the accumulation of conflicting changes that could destabilize the system.

Cognitive compounding therefore transforms incremental improvement into exponential effect. The system leverages repetition, reuse, and integration to scale the impact of small refinements. Each execution contributes to the refinement of the structure, and each refinement improves all future executions. The result is a system that increases its capability over time through the accumulation of precise, localized changes that propagate across its architecture.

Transferable Thinking

A system achieves transferability when its reasoning operates on structure rather than on surface content. Domains differ in language, context, and specific variables, but the underlying architecture of transformation remains consistent. Variables interact, constraints limit possible states, and sequences govern how change propagates. A system that encodes these elements at an abstract level can apply the same reasoning framework across different domains by remapping inputs into its existing structure. Advantage emerges because the system does not rebuild its thinking for each context. It reuses a stable architecture that adapts through translation rather than reconstruction.

Transfer begins with abstraction of variables. Instead of binding variables to domain-specific representations, the system defines them in terms of their functional role within a transformation. A variable may represent a resource, a constraint, a signal, or a state, independent of whether the domain is biological, financial, or mechanical. This abstraction allows new inputs to be mapped onto existing variable types. The system identifies what role each element plays rather than what it is called. Once mapped, the same relationships and constraints can be applied without modification to their structure.

Relationship invariance supports this mapping. The interactions between variables often follow consistent patterns across domains. Cause-and-effect chains, feedback loops, threshold effects, and dependency structures appear in different forms but share the same underlying logic. By encoding these patterns as reusable relationships, the system can apply them to new variable sets. This allows it to generate valid transformations in unfamiliar contexts because the structure of interaction remains consistent even when the content changes.

Constraint generalization maintains validity during transfer. Each domain has its own boundaries, but the concept of constraint remains constant. The system defines constraints as limits on variable states and transitions, then maps domain-specific limits into this framework. This ensures that transferred reasoning does not produce outputs that violate the rules of the new domain. Without this step, applying a model from one domain to another can generate states that are internally coherent but externally invalid.

Sequencing provides continuity. The order in which transformations occur often determines the outcome regardless of domain. By preserving sequencing logic, the system ensures that intermediate states are constructed correctly when applying its model to new inputs. This prevents the introduction of errors that arise from applying correct relationships in an incorrect order. Sequencing acts as a structural backbone that supports transfer across contexts.

Decomposition enables adaptation. When entering a new domain, the system breaks down complex inputs into components that can be mapped onto its existing structure. This process reveals which elements correspond to known variable types and which require new definitions. The system extends its model only where necessary, maintaining as much of its existing architecture as possible. This controlled adaptation preserves efficiency while expanding capability.

Feedback integration refines transfer. As the system applies its model in a new domain, it observes outcomes and compares them to predictions. Deviations indicate where the mapping between domains is incomplete or where relationships require adjustment. These refinements are integrated into the model, improving its ability to operate across contexts. Each successful transfer increases the system's capacity to generalize its reasoning.

Efficiency gains arise from reuse. A system that can transfer its thinking does not incur the cost of building a new model for each domain. It applies existing components, reducing the time and effort required to generate aligned outputs. This allows it to operate effectively in multiple contexts without a proportional increase in processing.

Error containment is preserved through structure. Because the system maintains defined variables, relationships, and constraints, errors introduced during transfer are localized to specific mappings or components. This allows for targeted correction without destabilizing the entire model. The system refines its transfer mechanism incrementally, improving accuracy while maintaining coherence.

Cross-domain advantage is therefore a function of structural consistency. A system that operates on abstracted variables, invariant relationships, and generalized constraints can apply its reasoning across different contexts with minimal modification. This allows it to produce aligned outputs in domains where others must rely on pattern recognition or rebuild their models from scratch.

Transferable thinking converts knowledge into a reusable framework. It enables the system to extend its capability beyond the domain in which it was developed, applying the same architecture to new problems. Over time, this creates a compounding advantage, as each successful transfer expands the system's ability to operate across a wider range of conditions while maintaining alignment with its underlying structure.

PART VIII

TRAINING THE LOGIC ENGINE

Chapter 23

Building Thinking Capacity

Thinking capacity is not defined by how much a system can process at once. It is defined by how well that processing is structured, preserved, and improved across repeated execution. Capacity increases when the system expands its ability to represent variables clearly, apply relationships accurately, enforce constraints consistently, and sequence transformations without loss of coherence. This expansion is architectural. It changes the internal organization of reasoning so that each unit of processing produces more aligned output and requires less correction.

The first layer of capacity is representation density. A system with low capacity handles inputs as coarse, undifferentiated signals, forcing it to operate with limited resolution. Increasing capacity requires decomposing inputs into finer variables with stable boundaries. Each additional variable increases the system's ability to distinguish between states, reducing ambiguity at the point of entry. This does not increase complexity for its own sake. It increases the precision with which the system can map inputs to its internal structure, allowing transformations to operate on clearly defined components.

Relationship depth follows representation. Once variables are defined, the system must encode how they interact across multiple conditions. Shallow models apply simple, often linear relationships that fail under variation. Increasing capacity requires layering relationships so that interactions can be evaluated under different states and constraints. This creates a network where changes propagate through multiple pathways, allowing the system to capture complex behavior without losing control over how transformations occur.

Constraint resolution stabilizes this network. As the number of variables and relationships increases, the number of possible states expands. Without constraints, the system cannot maintain alignment because it cannot distinguish valid states from invalid ones. Increasing capacity therefore involves defining tighter and more accurate boundaries on variables and transitions. These constraints reduce the state space to configurations that remain consistent with the model, allowing the system to operate at higher complexity without generating incoherent outputs.

Sequencing capacity determines how many transformations can be applied while preserving continuity. A system with limited capacity can only manage short sequences before losing track of intermediate states. Increasing capacity requires maintaining state across longer pathways, ensuring that each step builds correctly on the previous one. This involves tracking dependencies, preserving intermediate representations, and ensuring that transformations are applied in the correct order. As sequencing capacity increases, the system can handle more complex processes without breakdown.

Abstraction reduces the cost of increased capacity. As the system builds longer and more detailed pathways, it encapsulates stable sequences into reusable components. This allows complex transformations to be executed as single units within larger structures. Abstraction preserves the underlying logic while reducing the cognitive load required to apply it. This enables the system to expand its capacity without overwhelming its processing resources.

Feedback integration drives capacity growth. Each execution produces a comparison between predicted and observed outcomes, revealing where the model lacks precision. These deviations are localized and corrected, improving variable definitions, relationships, and constraints. As these refinements accumulate, the system's ability to represent and transform inputs improves. Capacity increases because the model becomes more accurate and efficient, reducing the need for corrective processing.

Error handling is part of capacity. A system with higher capacity does not eliminate error. It manages it more effectively. Errors are detected earlier, localized more precisely, and corrected with minimal impact on the rest of the model. This prevents the accumulation of inconsistencies that would otherwise reduce the system's ability to process new inputs.

Parallel processing extends capacity across multiple pathways. Independent sequences can be evaluated simultaneously, allowing the system to handle multiple transformations without increasing the depth of any single pathway. This increases throughput while maintaining the integrity of each sequence. The system identifies which components can operate independently and distributes processing accordingly.

Retention ensures that capacity gains persist. Improvements to variables, relationships, constraints, and sequences are integrated into the model so that future executions begin from an enhanced state. This prevents regression and allows the system to build on its previous refinements. Capacity is not rebuilt for each input. It is accumulated through continuous structural improvement.

Building thinking capacity is therefore a process of expanding and refining the architecture that governs reasoning. It increases the system's ability to handle complexity, maintain alignment, and produce consistent outputs across varying conditions. This expansion is controlled by structure, ensuring that each increase in capability is supported by clear definitions, stable relationships, enforced constraints, and organized sequences. Over time, the system becomes capable of processing more complex inputs with greater accuracy, reflecting the growth of its internal architecture rather than an increase in raw effort.

Daily Logic Training

Daily logic training increases capacity by repeatedly executing the same structured transformations until they become stable components of the system. The objective is not exposure to new ideas. It is the reinforcement and refinement of variable definition, relationship mapping, constraint enforcement, and sequencing under controlled conditions. Each session isolates a small set of components, applies them across multiple inputs, and integrates corrections directly into the model. Repetition stabilizes structure. Variation across inputs tests whether that structure holds under different conditions.

The training cycle begins with problem decomposition. Each input is reduced into explicit variables with defined boundaries. Ambiguous terms are converted into measurable or observable states. Hidden assumptions are surfaced and assigned to variables rather than left embedded in language. This step increases resolution at the point of entry and prevents downstream distortion. If the input cannot be decomposed cleanly, the system does not proceed. It refines definitions until the variables are stable.

Once variables are defined, relationships are constructed. The system specifies how changes in one variable alter the state of another, including direction, magnitude, and conditional dependencies. Nonlinear behavior is represented explicitly through thresholds or state-dependent rules rather than implied through intuition. The goal is to make interaction visible and testable. Relationships are not accepted because they sound plausible. They are encoded so that they can be executed and evaluated.

Constraints are then applied to limit the valid state space. Each variable is assigned bounds, and each relationship is checked against these bounds to ensure that transitions do not produce invalid states. Conflicts between constraints are resolved before execution. This step prevents the system from generating outputs that are internally consistent but externally impossible. Constraint clarity reduces the number of pathways that must be considered and increases the reliability of the remaining ones.

Sequencing follows. The system orders transformations so that intermediate states are constructed correctly. Dependencies are respected. Outputs from one step become inputs to the next without loss of definition. Where multiple sequences are possible, the system evaluates each for validity and selects the pathway that preserves constraints and minimizes unnecessary transformations. Sequencing errors are treated as structural faults, not minor mistakes, because they propagate through the entire chain.

Execution produces an output that can be compared against an expected or observed state. The comparison is not qualitative. It identifies specific deviations between predicted and actual variable states. Each deviation is traced back through the sequence to the component responsible. This localization step prevents global adjustments that degrade correct parts of the model. Corrections are applied only where the structure fails.

Integration converts each correction into a permanent change. Updated variable definitions, refined relationships, or adjusted constraints are incorporated into the model so that the same error does not recur. The system does not rely on remembering past mistakes. It encodes the correction into its structure. This is where training compounds. Each session leaves the model in a more precise state than before.

Variation across sessions tests robustness. The system applies the same structure to inputs that differ in surface content but share underlying patterns. Successful transfer indicates that the structure is correctly abstracted. Failure indicates that variables or relationships are too tightly bound to specific cases. The system adjusts abstraction levels to preserve transferability without losing precision.

Time allocation is controlled to maintain consistency. Short, focused sessions applied daily are more effective than irregular, extended sessions because they preserve continuity in the model. Each session builds directly on the previous one, allowing refinements to accumulate without decay. Gaps in execution reduce retention and require re-establishing structure before new improvements can be integrated.

Daily logic training therefore operates as a structured loop: decompose, map, constrain, sequence, execute, compare, correct, integrate. Each pass through the loop increases the precision and stability of the system. Over time, these incremental refinements produce a model that handles more complex inputs with less correction, reflecting an increase in capacity driven by consistent, structured practice.

Argument Analysis

Argument analysis converts a continuous stream of language into a structured sequence of variables and transformations that can be inspected, executed, and corrected. The system does not evaluate whether an argument sounds coherent. It extracts the components that generate the conclusion and reconstructs the pathway step by step. Each statement is treated as a potential variable definition, a relationship claim, or a constraint. The goal is to expose the internal architecture that produces the final output, allowing the system to test whether each transition preserves validity.

The process begins with segmentation. The argument is divided into discrete statements that can be mapped to specific roles within a reasoning chain. Some statements define variables, assigning properties or states to entities. Others assert relationships, describing how a change in one variable affects another. Some introduce constraints, limiting the range of possible states or transitions. The system separates these roles so that each component can be evaluated independently. Language that compresses multiple roles into a single sentence is expanded into explicit parts to prevent hidden assumptions from passing through unexamined.

Once segmented, variables are stabilized. Each term is assigned a consistent definition that remains fixed across the argument. If a term shifts meaning between statements, the system treats it as two distinct variables rather than allowing semantic drift. This prevents invalid transitions where a conclusion appears to follow but actually depends on a change in definition. Stable variables form the foundation of the analysis because every relationship and constraint depends on their consistency.

Relationships are then reconstructed explicitly. The system identifies the direction of influence between variables and the conditions under which that influence holds. If an argument claims that one state produces another, the system specifies the mechanism or rule that connects them. Unsupported transitions are flagged as gaps. The system does not fill these gaps with intuition. It marks them as missing components that must be supplied for the argument to remain valid.

Constraints are applied to evaluate whether the reconstructed pathway can produce the stated conclusion without violating boundaries. Each step is checked against known limits on variable states and transitions. If a step requires a variable to exceed its defined range or a relationship to operate outside its valid conditions, the pathway fails at that point. This prevents arguments from reaching correct conclusions through invalid intermediate states.

Sequencing verifies that the order of transformations preserves continuity. The system ensures that each step uses inputs that have been properly defined and produced by prior steps. If a conclusion depends on information that has not been established within the chain, the system identifies a sequencing error. This often appears as an implicit assumption or a skipped transformation that the argument relies on but does not state.

Error localization isolates the exact point where validity breaks. Rather than rejecting the entire argument, the system traces the pathway to the first invalid transition. This allows targeted correction. A variable definition may need refinement, a relationship may require additional conditions, or a constraint may have been misapplied. By isolating the failure point, the system preserves valid components while repairing only the defective parts.

Comparative analysis strengthens the model by evaluating alternative pathways. The system constructs different sequences that could connect the same variables and tests them against constraints and observed outcomes. This reveals whether the original argument represents the only valid pathway or one of several possibilities. It also exposes where the argument may have selected a pathway that appears plausible but is less consistent with the structure.

Integration follows correction. Adjustments to variables, relationships, or constraints are incorporated into the system so that similar arguments are processed with improved accuracy. Each analyzed argument contributes to refining the model, increasing its ability to detect structural faults and validate correct reasoning across different contexts.

Argument analysis therefore transforms reasoning from a surface-level narrative into a mechanical system of components and transitions. By decomposing, stabilizing, mapping, constraining, sequencing, and correcting, the system gains control over how conclusions are produced. This allows it to distinguish between arguments that arrive at correct outputs through valid structure and those that reach similar outputs through invalid or incomplete pathways, preserving alignment across all stages of reasoning.

Scenario Simulation Training

Scenario simulation training increases decision quality by executing structured reasoning before real-world constraints force action. The system constructs a defined environment, assigns variables with measurable states, and runs transformations forward to observe how those states evolve under different inputs. This is not imaginative projection. It is controlled execution of a model where each step follows explicit relationships and constraints. By resolving pathways in advance, the system reduces uncertainty at the point of action and limits the number of unknown transitions that must be processed in real time.

The process begins with state construction. The system defines the current condition using explicit variables rather than general descriptions. Each variable is assigned a range and a starting value that reflects the present environment. Missing variables are identified and either estimated with defined uncertainty or excluded with acknowledgement of their absence. This creates a bounded starting state that can be manipulated without ambiguity. If the initial state is unclear, the simulation will propagate that uncertainty through every subsequent step, so precision at this stage determines the reliability of the entire sequence.

Once the state is defined, relationships are applied to determine how changes propagate. The system specifies how each variable influences others, including direction, magnitude, and conditional behavior. Interactions are not assumed to be linear. Thresholds, saturation points, and feedback loops are encoded so that the simulation can represent non-uniform behavior. This allows the system to observe how small changes in input can produce disproportionate changes in output when certain conditions are met.

Constraint enforcement limits the simulation to valid pathways. Each transition is checked against boundaries that define what states are possible within the environment. If a transformation produces an invalid state, the pathway is rejected or corrected before continuing. This prevents the system from exploring trajectories that appear internally consistent but cannot occur in practice. Constraints also reduce the number of pathways that must be evaluated, focusing the simulation on states that remain viable.

Sequencing determines how the simulation unfolds over time. The system orders transformations so that each step builds on the previous state without introducing discontinuities. Dependencies are respected, ensuring that variables are updated only after the inputs required for their transformation are available. Multiple sequences can be constructed to represent different decision options. Each sequence is executed independently, producing a set of potential future states that can be compared.

Branching expands the simulation across alternative decisions. At defined points in the sequence, the system introduces different inputs and evaluates how each alters the trajectory. This creates a tree of possible outcomes rather than a single linear pathway. Each branch is tracked with its own state evolution, allowing the system to compare not only final outcomes but also the intermediate states that lead to them. This reveals where divergence occurs and which decisions produce stable or unstable trajectories.

Evaluation compares simulated outcomes against defined objectives and constraints. The system measures how closely each trajectory aligns with desired states while remaining within valid boundaries. Tradeoffs are made explicit. A pathway that optimizes one variable may degrade another, and the system must quantify these interactions rather than relying on general preference. This allows decisions to be selected based on structured comparison rather than intuition.

Feedback from real-world execution is used to refine the simulation. After a decision is implemented, observed outcomes are compared to simulated predictions. Deviations indicate where relationships were incomplete, constraints were misapplied, or variables were poorly defined. These discrepancies are integrated into the model, improving the accuracy of future simulations. Over time, the system reduces the gap between simulated and actual outcomes, increasing confidence in pre-executed pathways.

Time compression provides efficiency. By running multiple sequences in simulation, the system evaluates outcomes that would otherwise require extended real-world execution. This allows it to discard low-quality pathways before committing resources. The system does not eliminate uncertainty, but it reduces the number of unknowns that must be resolved during execution.

Scenario simulation training therefore converts decision-making into a preparatory process where pathways are constructed, tested, and refined before action occurs. Each simulation improves the structure of the model, allowing future scenarios to be evaluated with greater accuracy and speed. Over repeated cycles, the system develops the ability to anticipate state transitions, select higher-quality pathways, and execute decisions with reduced reliance on real-time correction.

Chapter 24

Cognitive Discipline

Cognitive discipline is the enforcement layer that maintains structural integrity during reasoning. It does not expand what the system knows. It controls how the system is allowed to operate. Without discipline, variables drift, relationships are applied inconsistently, constraints are bypassed, and sequencing breaks under pressure. The system may still produce outputs, but those outputs are no longer traceable to a stable architecture. Discipline prevents this degradation by forcing every transformation to remain within defined rules, even when speed, emotion, or external pressure would otherwise override them.

The first function of discipline is variable control. Each variable must retain a fixed definition across the entire reasoning process. When a term begins to shift meaning to support a conclusion, discipline halts the process and forces redefinition. This prevents the system from reaching conclusions through semantic substitution. Variable control also requires that all relevant variables are made explicit before transformation begins. Hidden variables introduce uncontrolled influence, leading to outputs that cannot be traced back to defined inputs.

Relationship enforcement follows. Once variables are defined, the system must apply relationships consistently. A relationship that holds under one condition cannot be selectively ignored when it produces an inconvenient result. Discipline ensures that all transformations follow the same rules regardless of outcome preference. This prevents the system from altering its internal logic to maintain coherence with a desired conclusion.

Constraint adherence limits the system to valid states. Constraints define the boundaries within which variables can exist and interact. Under pressure, there is a tendency to relax these boundaries to reach a conclusion more quickly. Discipline prevents this by requiring that every intermediate state be checked against defined limits. If a pathway violates a constraint, it is rejected regardless of how efficient or appealing it appears. This preserves alignment with reality and prevents the accumulation of invalid states.

Sequencing integrity ensures that transformations occur in the correct order. Skipping steps or rearranging sequences to accelerate output introduces errors that propagate through the system. Discipline enforces the requirement that each step must be completed and validated before proceeding. Dependencies are respected, and intermediate states are preserved. This maintains continuity across the reasoning chain and prevents the introduction of hidden assumptions.

Attention allocation is regulated to prevent fragmentation. A system with undisciplined attention shifts between variables and pathways without completing any of them, leading to partial processing and unresolved states. Discipline constrains attention to a defined pathway until it is executed and evaluated. Parallel processing is only allowed when pathways are independent and fully specified. This prevents interference between sequences and preserves clarity.

Error handling is governed by discipline. When a deviation is detected, the system does not ignore it or compensate with additional transformations. It stops and localizes the source of the error. Corrections are applied at the point of failure rather than downstream. This prevents the accumulation of layered adjustments that obscure the original structure. Discipline treats errors as structural faults that must be resolved before further processing continues.

Consistency across executions reinforces discipline. The same input must produce the same output when processed through the same structure. If outputs vary, the system identifies where inconsistency has been introduced. This may occur through variable drift, relationship misapplication, or constraint violation. Discipline requires that these inconsistencies be resolved so that the system remains predictable and repeatable.

Resistance to external pressure is a critical component. Social influence, time constraints, and emotional responses all introduce forces that push the system toward faster or more convenient outputs. Discipline acts as a buffer, maintaining adherence to structure despite these pressures. The system does not accelerate by removing steps or relaxing rules. It accelerates only when its structure becomes more efficient through refinement.

Cognitive discipline therefore maintains the integrity of the reasoning architecture. It ensures that every transformation is traceable, every variable is stable, every relationship is applied consistently, and every constraint is enforced. Over time, this produces a system that generates reliable outputs under a wide range of conditions because its operation is governed by structure rather than by fluctuation in input or context.

Removing Emotional Defaults

Emotional defaults are preloaded response patterns that alter variable selection, relationship weighting, and constraint enforcement before structured reasoning begins. They operate as automatic transformations applied at the input layer, shaping how the system interprets a situation before it has defined the variables involved. This introduces bias at the earliest stage of processing, which then propagates through every subsequent step. Stabilizing output requires intercepting these transformations, isolating their effect, and preventing them from modifying the structure that governs reasoning.

The process begins with detection at the input boundary. When an input enters the system, the initial interpretation often includes affective tagging such as threat, reward, urgency, or aversion. These tags shift attention, amplify certain variables, and suppress others. The system must separate the raw input from these tags by explicitly reconstructing the state in neutral terms. Variables are defined based on observable properties rather than on how the input is perceived. This prevents emotional weighting from determining which components are included in the model.

Once variables are stabilized, relationship weighting is examined. Emotional defaults tend to exaggerate specific pathways, increasing the perceived strength or immediacy of certain interactions. For example, a low-probability negative outcome may be treated as dominant, altering the sequence of transformations. The system recalibrates these relationships by assigning weights based on defined conditions and measurable likelihoods rather than perceived intensity. This restores proportional influence across the model.

Constraint enforcement is then restored. Emotional pressure often leads to the relaxation or selective application of constraints, allowing invalid states to be considered because they align with a preferred outcome. The system reasserts boundaries by checking each transformation against fixed limits. Any pathway that requires a violation of these limits is removed, regardless of its emotional appeal. This ensures that outputs remain within valid state space.

Sequencing is protected from compression. Emotional urgency drives the system to skip intermediate steps and move directly to conclusions. This introduces hidden assumptions and breaks continuity in the reasoning chain. The system enforces full sequencing, requiring that each transformation be executed and validated in order. This prevents the insertion of unverified transitions that would otherwise destabilize the output.

Attention is redistributed to maintain coverage. Emotional defaults narrow focus onto a subset of variables while excluding others that may be critical for accurate modeling. The system expands attention back to the full set of defined variables, ensuring that no component is omitted due to its lack of emotional salience. This maintains completeness in the representation of the state.

Output stabilization emerges from consistency in structure. When variables are defined neutrally, relationships are weighted proportionally, constraints are enforced uniformly, and sequencing is preserved, the system produces outputs that are independent of transient emotional states. The same input yields the same output regardless of internal fluctuations because the processing pathway remains unchanged.

Feedback integration further reduces emotional influence. When actual outcomes are compared to predictions, discrepancies reveal where emotional weighting distorted the model. These discrepancies are traced to specific components and corrected. Over time, the system reduces the influence of emotional defaults because they consistently produce deviations from observed states.

Removing emotional defaults does not eliminate affective signals. It isolates them from structural processing. Emotional responses can still be represented as variables within the model, allowing their effects to be evaluated explicitly rather than implicitly shaping the entire pathway. This preserves their informational value without allowing them to override the architecture.

Stabilizing output therefore depends on maintaining separation between perception and processing. Inputs are translated into defined variables before any transformation occurs. Relationships, constraints, and sequences operate on this structured representation without interference from automatic weighting. The result is a system that produces consistent, traceable outputs, where variation arises from changes in input conditions rather than from internal fluctuation in how those inputs are processed.

Rewriting Thinking Patterns

Thinking patterns are persistent model fragments that determine how variables are defined, how relationships are constructed, and how constraints are applied before conscious reasoning begins. They are not isolated habits. They are embedded structures that execute automatically, producing consistent transformations across different inputs. When a pattern is flawed, it introduces the same distortion repeatedly, regardless of context. Rewriting thinking patterns requires identifying the structural error within the model, removing the faulty component, and replacing it with a configuration that produces valid state transitions under repeated execution.

The process begins with failure detection across multiple instances. A single incorrect output does not confirm a flawed pattern. The system looks for repeated deviations where different inputs produce errors that share the same structural signature. These signatures often appear as consistent misclassification of variables, incorrect direction of influence in relationships, or systematic relaxation of constraints. By isolating what remains constant across failures, the system identifies the underlying component responsible for the distortion rather than focusing on the surface-level differences between cases.

Once identified, the flawed component is extracted from the model. This requires isolating the exact transformation that produces the error. The system traces the reasoning chain backward from the incorrect output to the point where a variable was misdefined, a relationship was incorrectly applied, or a constraint was bypassed. This component is removed from active use. It is not suppressed temporarily. It is treated as invalid within the model so that it cannot be reintroduced during subsequent processing.

Replacement requires constructing a corrected component that performs the same functional role without producing invalid states. If the flaw originated in variable definition, the system refines the boundaries of that variable so that it remains stable across contexts. If the flaw originated in a relationship, the system specifies the correct conditions under which the interaction holds, including direction, magnitude, and limitations. If the flaw originated in constraint handling, the system redefines the boundaries and ensures that they are enforced uniformly across all pathways.

Integration embeds the corrected component into the model so that it becomes the default transformation in future executions. This step is critical because without integration, the system may revert to the previous pattern under pressure or when processing unfamiliar inputs. The corrected component must be applied repeatedly across different contexts to ensure that it produces valid outputs consistently. This repetition stabilizes the new pattern and replaces the previous one at the architectural level.

Conflict resolution ensures that the new component does not introduce inconsistencies with existing parts of the model. The system evaluates how the replacement interacts with other variables, relationships, and constraints. If conflicts arise, additional adjustments are made to maintain coherence. This prevents the accumulation of localized fixes that destabilize the overall structure.

Reinforcement occurs through repeated execution under varied conditions. The system applies the new pattern across inputs that differ in surface characteristics but share underlying structure. Successful execution across these cases confirms that the pattern has been generalized correctly. Failures are used to refine the component further until it operates reliably.

Suppression of the old pattern is achieved through disuse and structural invalidation. When the corrected component consistently produces valid outputs, the system no longer has a functional need for the previous pattern. Over time, the pathways associated with the flawed component are no longer activated, reducing the likelihood of regression.

Rewriting thinking patterns therefore operates as a controlled replacement of structural components within the reasoning architecture. It does not rely on intention or awareness alone. It requires explicit identification of the faulty transformation, construction of a valid alternative, and integration of that alternative into the system so that it governs future processing. Over time, this process shifts the system's default behavior, producing outputs that remain aligned across different inputs because the underlying structure has been corrected.

Internal Consistency and External Alignment

Internal consistency refers to whether the system's variables, relationships, constraints, and sequences operate without contradiction. External alignment refers to whether those same components produce state transitions that match observable conditions. A system can satisfy one without the other. It can remain internally coherent while drifting away from reality, or it can match isolated observations while relying on unstable internal structure. Maintaining structure requires both to operate simultaneously. Internal consistency preserves the integrity of transformations. External alignment anchors those transformations to valid outcomes.

The process begins with variable stability. Each variable must retain a fixed definition across all pathways so that transformations operate on the same underlying entity. Internal consistency fails when a variable shifts meaning between steps, allowing a conclusion to follow from a different definition than the one originally used. External alignment fails when a variable's definition does not correspond to observable states. The system enforces stability by locking definitions and validating them against measurable conditions. If a variable cannot be observed or inferred with defined bounds, it is either refined or removed from the model.

Relationship coherence maintains internal structure. Each relationship must produce the same directional effect under the same conditions across all pathways. If a relationship changes behavior depending on the desired outcome, the system loses consistency. External alignment requires that these relationships produce state changes that match observed interactions. The system tests each relationship by executing it across different inputs and comparing the resulting states to real outcomes. Relationships that fail this test are modified or replaced.

Constraint enforcement ensures that all transformations remain within valid boundaries. Internally, constraints prevent the system from generating states that contradict its own definitions. Externally, they ensure that those states remain possible within the environment being modeled. When constraints are inconsistently applied, the system may produce outputs that appear correct but rely on intermediate states that cannot exist. The system enforces constraints at each step, rejecting pathways that violate boundaries regardless of their apparent efficiency.

Sequencing integrity connects internal consistency with external alignment. Each transformation must occur in an order that reflects how state changes propagate in reality. Internally, sequencing ensures that each step uses properly defined inputs from prior steps. Externally, it ensures that the order of operations matches the causal structure of the environment. Errors in sequencing often produce outputs that appear coherent but fail when executed because the underlying transitions were applied out of order.

Feedback integration binds the two layers together. After execution, the system compares predicted states to observed outcomes. Internal consistency is evaluated by checking whether the reasoning chain contained contradictions or undefined transitions. External alignment is evaluated by measuring how closely the predicted states match reality. Deviations are traced to specific components, allowing targeted correction. This process continuously adjusts the model so that both internal structure and external correspondence improve together.

Drift occurs when one layer is maintained without the other. A system that prioritizes internal consistency alone can refine its structure while becoming detached from reality. A system that prioritizes external alignment without internal consistency may match outcomes in isolated cases but lacks a stable framework for generalization. Maintaining structure requires balancing both, ensuring that each refinement preserves coherence while improving correspondence with observed states.

Scalability depends on this balance. As the system expands to handle more variables and more complex relationships, internal consistency prevents collapse under complexity, while external alignment ensures that increased complexity produces valid outputs. Without both, the system cannot extend its capability without introducing instability.

Maintaining structure therefore requires continuous enforcement of consistency within the model and continuous validation against the environment. Each variable, relationship, constraint, and sequence must satisfy both conditions. Over time, this dual enforcement produces a system that generates outputs that are not only internally coherent but also reliably aligned with the states they are intended to represent.

Chapter 25

Continuous Evolution

Continuous evolution is the process by which a system maintains and improves its reasoning architecture through repeated exposure to inputs, execution of transformations, and integration of feedback. The system does not reach a fixed state of completion. It remains in an adaptive loop where each execution has the potential to refine variables, relationships, constraints, and sequencing. Stability is not achieved by freezing the model. It is achieved by preserving structural integrity while allowing controlled modification of its components.

The process begins with persistent exposure to variation. A system that operates on a narrow range of inputs cannot detect the limits of its structure. Variation introduces conditions where existing relationships are tested outside their usual range, revealing where definitions are too broad, too narrow, or incorrectly applied. These conditions generate deviations between predicted and observed states, providing the signal required for refinement. Without variation, the system may appear stable while containing latent structural errors that only emerge under different inputs.

Detection of deviation drives change. Each execution produces a comparison between expected outcomes and actual results. The system measures these differences at the level of individual variables and transitions rather than at the level of final output alone. This granular comparison allows the system to identify which component of the model failed to produce the correct state. Broad comparisons obscure the source of error and lead to ineffective adjustments. Precision in detection is required for targeted modification.

Localization isolates the component responsible for deviation. The system traces the reasoning chain to the point where the predicted state diverges from the observed state. This may occur due to incorrect variable definition, incomplete relationship mapping, or improper constraint enforcement. By isolating the exact point of failure, the system avoids modifying components that are already functioning correctly. This preserves stability while enabling focused refinement.

Modification adjusts the identified component to produce a corrected transformation. Variable definitions are refined to better match observable states. Relationships are updated to reflect accurate direction, magnitude, and conditional behavior. Constraints are recalibrated to ensure that valid states are included and invalid states are excluded. These modifications are applied with minimal scope, altering only what is necessary to resolve the deviation.

Integration embeds the modification into the system's architecture. The corrected component becomes the default for future executions, ensuring that the same deviation does not recur. Integration distinguishes evolution from temporary adjustment. Without it, the system would need to rediscover the same correction repeatedly, preventing accumulation of improvement.

Validation confirms that the modification does not introduce new inconsistencies. The system re-executes pathways that depend on the modified component, checking for unintended effects on other variables, relationships, or constraints. If conflicts arise, additional adjustments are made until coherence is restored. This step maintains internal consistency while improving external alignment.

Iteration repeats the cycle. Each new input provides additional data, generating new opportunities for refinement. The system accumulates these modifications over time, gradually increasing the precision and reliability of its model. The rate of evolution depends on the frequency of feedback and the system's ability to integrate corrections without destabilizing existing structure.

Retention ensures that improvements persist across time. The system stores refined components in a way that they are consistently applied in future executions. This prevents regression and allows the system to build on prior refinements. Retention converts individual corrections into long-term capability.

Continuous evolution therefore operates as a controlled feedback loop where the system detects deviation, isolates its source, modifies the relevant component, and integrates the correction into its architecture. This process allows the system to adapt to changing conditions while maintaining structural integrity. Over time, the accumulation of precise modifications produces a model that remains aligned with the environment across a wide range of inputs, reflecting an architecture that improves through use rather than one that remains static.

Rapid Belief Updating

Rapid belief updating is the system's ability to modify its internal model at the point where new data conflicts with existing structure, without destabilizing the rest of the architecture. A belief is not treated as a static idea. It is a component of the model that encodes a variable definition, a relationship, or a constraint. When incoming information produces a state that the current model cannot generate, the system does not preserve the belief and reinterpret the data. It modifies the component responsible for the mismatch so that future executions produce aligned states.

The process begins with mismatch detection. Each execution produces a predicted state based on current variables and relationships. Observed data is then compared to this predicted state at the level of individual variables rather than at the level of general outcome. A difference between predicted and observed values signals that at least one component of the model is misaligned. The system measures the magnitude and location of this difference, identifying whether it originates from incorrect input representation, faulty relationships, or constraint misapplication.

Localization isolates the belief that generated the error. The system traces the transformation chain backward to the first point where the predicted state diverges from the observed state. This point corresponds to a specific component. A variable may be defined too broadly, allowing states that do not occur. A relationship may assume a direction or magnitude that does not hold under the current conditions. A constraint may exclude valid states or allow invalid ones. By identifying the exact component, the system avoids modifying unrelated parts of the model.

Replacement modifies the component to resolve the mismatch. If a variable is misdefined, its boundaries are tightened or expanded to reflect observed states. If a relationship is incorrect, its conditions are specified more precisely, including where it holds and where it fails. If a constraint is inaccurate, its limits are recalibrated. The modification is minimal. It changes only what is required to align predictions with observations, preserving the rest of the structure.

Integration embeds the updated component into the model so that future predictions incorporate the correction. This step ensures that the system does not need to reprocess the same mismatch repeatedly. The updated belief becomes part of the architecture, influencing all subsequent executions that depend on that component. Integration converts a single correction into a persistent change in behavior.

Speed is determined by how directly the system can perform this sequence. A system with high adaptive capacity detects mismatch early, localizes the error precisely, and applies a targeted modification without affecting unrelated components. Delay occurs when mismatch detection is coarse, localization is imprecise, or modifications are applied broadly, requiring additional corrections to restore stability. Rapid updating therefore depends on resolution at each stage of the process.

Stability is maintained by constraint checking during integration. Each modification is tested against existing components to ensure that it does not introduce contradictions. If a change to one relationship conflicts with another, the system resolves the conflict before proceeding. This prevents the accumulation of incompatible adjustments that would degrade the model's coherence.

Iteration refines the update. After integration, the system re-executes the pathway under the same and varied conditions to confirm that the modification produces consistent alignment. If residual deviations remain, additional adjustments are made. This iterative process ensures that the updated belief operates correctly across different inputs rather than only resolving a single instance.

Retention ensures persistence. The updated component is stored as the default transformation for future executions. The system does not rely on recalling that a belief was incorrect. It replaces the incorrect structure so that it is no longer used. This prevents regression and supports continuous adaptation.

Rapid belief updating therefore operates as a controlled modification of the system's internal architecture in response to new data. It maintains alignment by treating beliefs as adjustable components rather than fixed truths. Each update improves the model's ability to generate accurate states, allowing the system to adapt to changing conditions while preserving the integrity of its overall structure.

Using Failure as Data

Failure provides information about where the system's structure fails to produce valid state transitions. It is not treated as a terminal outcome. It is treated as a measurement of deviation between predicted and observed states. Each failure contains a signal that identifies which component of the model produced an incorrect transformation. The system extracts this signal and uses it to refine variables, relationships, constraints, or sequencing so that the same pathway produces a different result under the same conditions.

The process begins with precise comparison. The system does not evaluate failure at the level of general outcome. It decomposes both the predicted and observed states into their underlying variables and measures the difference at each point. This reveals whether the failure originates from incorrect input representation, inaccurate transformation, or constraint violation. Without this decomposition, the system cannot determine where the model diverged from reality.

Localization isolates the structural fault. The system traces the reasoning sequence backward to the first point where the predicted state deviates from the observed state. This point corresponds to a specific transformation. A variable may have been defined with incorrect boundaries, allowing a state that does not occur. A relationship may have been applied outside of its valid conditions. A constraint may have been ignored or incorrectly set. Identifying this point prevents the system from applying broad corrections that affect components that are already functioning correctly.

Reconstruction replaces the faulty transformation. The system modifies the identified component so that it produces a state closer to the observed outcome. Variable definitions are adjusted to reflect actual ranges. Relationships are refined to include correct direction, magnitude, and conditions. Constraints are recalibrated to include valid states and exclude invalid ones. This reconstruction is minimal in scope, targeting only the component responsible for the failure.

Validation ensures that the correction resolves the failure without introducing new inconsistencies. The system re-executes the pathway using the modified component and compares the resulting state to the observed outcome. It also evaluates other pathways that depend on the same component to confirm that they remain valid. If new deviations appear, additional adjustments are made until coherence is restored.

Integration embeds the correction into the model. The updated component becomes the default for future executions, preventing the same failure from recurring. This step converts the failure from a one-time event into a permanent improvement in the system's structure. Without integration, the system would need to rediscover the correction repeatedly.

Aggregation of failures reveals patterns. When multiple failures are analyzed, the system identifies recurring structural weaknesses. These may appear as consistent misdefinition of certain variables, repeated misapplication of specific relationships, or systematic relaxation of constraints under certain conditions. Addressing these patterns produces larger improvements than correcting individual failures in isolation.

Error magnitude influences priority. Failures that produce large deviations are addressed first because they indicate components that significantly distort the model. Smaller deviations are addressed after major structural issues are resolved. This prioritization ensures that resources are allocated to corrections that produce the greatest improvement in alignment.

Feedback timing affects efficiency. Immediate analysis of failure allows the system to localize the fault while the reasoning sequence is still accessible. Delayed analysis increases the difficulty of tracing the error because intermediate states may no longer be available. Rapid integration of corrections improves the system's ability to adapt in real time.

Using failure as data therefore transforms error into a mechanism for structural refinement. Each failure provides a measurable indication of where the model diverges from reality. By decomposing, localizing, reconstructing, validating, and integrating, the system converts these deviations into improvements in its architecture. Over time, this process reduces the frequency and magnitude of failure, producing outputs that remain aligned across a wider range of conditions because the underlying structure has been continuously corrected.

Building an Internal Intelligence System

An internal intelligence system is defined by its ability to generate, test, and modify its own structure without relying on external correction for each adjustment. It operates as a closed-loop architecture where inputs are translated into variables, processed through defined relationships and constraints, and evaluated against observed outcomes, with each cycle producing modifications that are retained and applied to future executions. Intelligence in this context is not a property of stored information. It is a property of how the system reorganizes itself when its outputs fail to match the environment.

The system begins with a stable representational layer. Inputs are decomposed into variables with fixed definitions and bounded states so that transformations operate on consistent components. Without this layer, corrections cannot be localized because the system lacks a fixed reference for what each element represents. Representation must be precise enough to distinguish meaningful differences in state, but constrained enough to prevent uncontrolled expansion of variables that would dilute the model.

Transformation logic forms the second layer. Relationships between variables are encoded as executable rules that determine how state changes propagate. These rules include direction of influence, magnitude under different conditions, and the presence of feedback loops that alter behavior over time. The system does not treat these relationships as static. It evaluates them continuously through execution, using discrepancies between predicted and observed states to determine where the rules fail to produce accurate transitions.

Constraint enforcement stabilizes the architecture. Each variable and transformation is limited by boundaries that define valid states and transitions. These constraints prevent the system from generating outputs that are internally consistent but externally impossible. Enforcement occurs at every step of processing, ensuring that invalid states are rejected immediately rather than carried forward and compounded. This containment preserves coherence as the system evolves.

The feedback layer connects output to modification. After each execution, the system compares predicted states to observed outcomes at the level of individual variables. Differences are measured, localized, and traced back to the specific component responsible. This creates a direct mapping between error and structure, allowing the system to identify exactly where modification is required. Feedback is not treated as a general signal of success or failure. It is decomposed into actionable data that targets specific elements of the model.

Modification mechanisms adjust the identified components. Variable definitions are refined to better match observed states. Relationships are updated to reflect accurate interaction patterns. Constraints are recalibrated to include valid states and exclude invalid ones. These adjustments are applied with minimal scope to avoid disrupting components that already produce correct transformations. Each modification is evaluated for its effect on both local pathways and the broader architecture.

Integration ensures persistence of change. Once a modification is validated, it is incorporated into the model so that future executions use the updated structure by default. This prevents the system from reverting to previous configurations and allows improvements to accumulate over time. Integration converts individual corrections into systemic capability.

Self-monitoring extends the system's control over its own operation. The system tracks consistency across executions, detecting when identical inputs produce different outputs or when similar structures yield divergent results. These inconsistencies indicate instability within the architecture. The system isolates the source and applies corrective adjustments to restore repeatability. This monitoring function maintains reliability as the model grows in complexity.

Scalability emerges from modular organization. As the system expands, it encapsulates stable sequences of transformations into reusable components. These modules can be applied across different pathways without redefinition, increasing efficiency while preserving structure. Modularization allows the system to handle larger and more complex inputs without increasing the risk of structural breakdown.

An internal intelligence system therefore operates as a self-correcting architecture where each execution contributes to its refinement. It maintains stable representation, enforces constraints, evaluates outcomes against predictions, and integrates targeted modifications. Over time, this process produces a system that improves through use, generating outputs that remain aligned with the environment because its structure is continuously adjusted to reflect the conditions under which it operates.

PART IX

THE FUTURE OF THINKING

Chapter 26

The New Intellectual Class

A new intellectual class forms when advantage shifts from possession of information to control over how information is structured, transformed, and applied. The defining feature is not access. Information is widely available and increasingly uniform across participants. Differentiation emerges from the architecture that processes it. Individuals operating with structured reasoning systems produce consistent, high-quality outputs from the same inputs that others process into noise. The divide is therefore structural. It separates systems that maintain stable variables, enforce relationships, and integrate feedback from systems that operate through approximation and inconsistency.

This class is defined by control over representation. Inputs are not accepted at face value. They are decomposed into variables with explicit boundaries before any transformation occurs. This prevents ambiguity from entering the system and ensures that all subsequent processing operates on stable components. Systems without this control inherit the ambiguity of their inputs, leading to outputs that vary depending on interpretation rather than structure. The ability to stabilize representation creates a consistent starting point across different contexts.

Transformation capability distinguishes performance within the class. Structured systems apply relationships that are defined, testable, and condition-dependent. They can map how changes propagate across variables and predict intermediate states before execution. This allows them to evaluate multiple pathways and select those that remain within constraints while optimizing for desired outcomes. Systems without this capability rely on pattern recognition and surface similarity, which fail as complexity increases or when inputs deviate from familiar forms.

Constraint enforcement separates valid outputs from plausible ones. Members of this class operate within defined boundaries, rejecting pathways that violate constraints even when those pathways appear efficient or intuitive. This produces outputs that remain stable under execution because they are generated within valid state space. Systems that do not enforce constraints produce outputs that may appear correct but collapse when applied because they rely on intermediate states that cannot exist.

Feedback integration sustains advantage over time. Structured systems treat each execution as a source of data, measuring deviations and modifying their architecture accordingly. This continuous refinement increases precision and reduces error across repeated use. Systems that do not integrate feedback remain static, repeating the same transformations regardless of outcome. Over time, the gap between adaptive and static systems widens because one accumulates structural improvements while the other does not.

Consistency across execution defines reliability. The same input processed through the same structure produces the same output. This repeatability allows for scaling because results can be predicted and reproduced. Systems that lack consistency produce variable outputs, making them difficult to trust or extend. Reliability becomes a direct function of structural stability rather than individual effort.

Transferability expands the scope of application. Members of this class operate on abstracted variables and invariant relationships, allowing them to apply their reasoning architecture across domains. They do not rebuild their models for each new context. They map new inputs onto existing structures, reducing the cost of adaptation and increasing speed of alignment. This creates an advantage in environments where conditions change and new domains must be understood quickly.

Speed emerges from structure rather than from compression. As the system refines its architecture, it reduces unnecessary transformations and eliminates invalid pathways earlier in the sequence. This allows it to produce outputs faster without sacrificing accuracy. Systems that prioritize speed without structure achieve throughput by bypassing steps, which increases error and reduces reliability. Structured systems achieve speed by improving the organization of their processing.

The boundary between classes becomes visible in output quality over time. Initially, differences may appear minimal because both structured and unstructured systems can produce acceptable results in simple conditions. As complexity increases and sequences extend, structural differences produce divergence. One system maintains alignment, while the other accumulates error. This divergence is not sudden. It is the result of compounding differences in how each system processes information.

The new intellectual class therefore consists of systems that operate with controlled, self-correcting architecture. Their advantage is not based on what they know, but on how they transform what they know into consistent, aligned outputs. Over time, this structural advantage compounds, producing a widening gap between those who can maintain alignment across complex conditions and those who cannot.

The Cognitive Divide

The cognitive divide emerges from differences in how systems are built, not from differences in how much information they hold. Two systems can operate on the same inputs and produce outputs that diverge because their internal architecture processes those inputs differently. One system stabilizes variables, enforces relationships, and constrains transitions. The other allows ambiguity, substitutes patterns for structure, and relaxes boundaries under pressure. The result is inequality at the level of transformation. Output quality becomes a function of structure rather than access, and that difference compounds over time.

The divide begins at the level of representation. A structured system decomposes inputs into explicit variables with defined boundaries, allowing it to operate on stable components. An unstructured system processes inputs as undifferentiated signals, relying on surface interpretation that shifts with context. This creates inconsistency at the point of entry. The same input can be interpreted differently across instances, producing variability before any reasoning occurs. The structured system maintains a fixed starting state. The unstructured system does not, and this instability propagates through every subsequent step.

Relationship handling widens the gap. Structured systems encode how variables interact under specific conditions, allowing them to predict how changes propagate across the model. Unstructured systems substitute pattern recognition, applying associations that worked in previous cases without verifying whether the underlying conditions are the same. This produces acceptable outputs in familiar environments but fails when inputs deviate. The difference is not visible in simple scenarios. It becomes pronounced as the number of variables and interactions increases.

Constraint enforcement separates valid outputs from plausible ones. Structured systems restrict transformations to states that remain within defined boundaries, preventing invalid pathways from entering the sequence. Unstructured systems often bypass constraints when they conflict with intuitive conclusions, allowing outputs that appear coherent but cannot be executed in reality. These invalid states accumulate, creating divergence that is not immediately visible but becomes significant over time.

Sequencing integrity determines whether transformations maintain continuity. Structured systems preserve the order of operations, ensuring that each step builds on a correctly formed intermediate state. Unstructured systems compress sequences, skipping steps or rearranging transformations to reach conclusions more quickly. This introduces hidden assumptions and breaks the chain of causality. The outputs may still appear correct in isolated cases, but they lack the structural support required for consistent reproduction.

Feedback integration drives separation across time. Structured systems measure deviations between predicted and observed states, localize errors, and modify their architecture. Each execution contributes to refinement, increasing accuracy and efficiency. Unstructured systems either ignore feedback or apply it inconsistently, often adjusting conclusions without correcting the underlying model. This prevents accumulation of improvement. Over repeated cycles, one system evolves while the other remains static or degrades.

Consistency creates reliability. A structured system produces the same output from the same input because its architecture is stable. This allows it to scale, as results can be predicted and extended across contexts. An unstructured system produces variable outputs because its processing depends on transient factors such as interpretation, context, or internal state. This variability limits its ability to operate under increased complexity or to maintain performance across domains.

Access to opportunity is shaped by this divide. Systems that maintain alignment can evaluate complex scenarios, identify valid pathways, and execute decisions with predictable outcomes. Systems that lack structure operate with higher error rates and greater uncertainty, limiting their ability to engage with complex environments. The inequality is not imposed externally. It emerges from differences in how each system processes information.

The cognitive divide therefore reflects a structural inequality in reasoning architecture. It is defined by the presence or absence of stable variables, coherent relationships, enforced constraints, and consistent sequencing. Over time, these differences produce divergence in output quality, adaptability, and reliability. The gap widens not because one system has more information, but because one system continuously refines how it uses that information while the other does not.

Logic as Dominant Skill

Logic becomes dominant when it governs how inputs are transformed into outputs across all domains, controlling variable definition, relationship mapping, constraint enforcement, and sequencing without relying on context-specific heuristics. It operates as the central architecture through which all information passes, determining whether a system produces stable, repeatable results or variable, context-dependent outcomes. Advantage emerges because logic standardizes transformation. It removes dependence on familiarity and replaces it with a consistent process that can be applied to any input that can be decomposed into structured components.

The system begins by stabilizing variables. Logic enforces that each element of an input is defined with fixed boundaries before transformation occurs. This prevents ambiguity from propagating through the model and ensures that every subsequent operation acts on the same underlying representation. Without this control, the same input can produce different outputs because the variables shift between interpretations. Logic removes this variability by locking definitions at the point of entry.

Relationship mapping follows, where logic specifies how variables interact under defined conditions. These interactions are not inferred from similarity to previous cases. They are constructed based on explicit rules that can be executed and tested. This allows the system to predict how changes in one variable will affect others across different states. As the number of variables increases, this structured mapping prevents the exponential growth of possible pathways from overwhelming the system, because invalid transitions are eliminated early.

Constraint enforcement defines the limits within which the system can operate. Logic restricts transformations to states that remain valid, rejecting any pathway that violates defined boundaries. This ensures that outputs are not only internally consistent but also executable within the environment. Systems that lack this enforcement may produce outputs that appear correct but rely on intermediate states that cannot exist. Logic prevents these pathways from being considered, maintaining alignment with reality.

Sequencing organizes transformations into coherent chains. Each step is executed in an order that preserves dependencies and maintains continuity of state. Logic prevents compression of sequences that would skip necessary transformations, ensuring that conclusions are derived from fully constructed pathways. This preserves traceability, allowing the system to identify exactly how an output was produced and where adjustments must be made if errors occur.

Feedback integration strengthens logic as a dominant skill. Each execution produces data that can be compared to predicted states. Deviations are localized and used to refine variables, relationships, and constraints. This continuous adjustment improves the system's accuracy over time, allowing logic to operate with increasing precision across a wider range of conditions. Systems that do not integrate feedback remain fixed, limiting their ability to adapt.

Transferability extends the advantage across domains. Because logic operates on abstracted structures rather than domain-specific content, it can be applied to new contexts by mapping inputs onto existing variable types and relationships. This allows the system to generate aligned outputs in unfamiliar environments without rebuilding its architecture. The same reasoning process scales across different problems, increasing efficiency and reducing the cost of adaptation.

Efficiency emerges from elimination of unnecessary transformations. Logic identifies pathways that do not contribute to valid state changes and removes them from the sequence. This reduces processing time while maintaining accuracy. The system becomes faster not by bypassing steps, but by improving the organization of its operations so that only necessary transformations are executed.

Reliability is the final effect. A system governed by logic produces consistent outputs from consistent inputs, maintains alignment under variation, and improves through feedback. This reliability allows it to operate at scale, handle complexity, and maintain performance across different conditions.

Logic therefore functions as the primary advantage because it defines how all information is processed. It controls the structure of reasoning, ensuring that outputs remain aligned, repeatable, and adaptable. Over time, this control produces a compounding effect, where each refinement to the logical structure improves all future processing, creating a system that increases its capability through the continuous application of structured transformation.

Reclaiming Human Thought

Reclaiming human thought requires rebuilding the internal architecture that governs how inputs are converted into decisions. The system must be restructured at the level of variable definition, relationship mapping, constraint enforcement, and sequencing so that each transformation produces a valid state transition. Modern environments supply high volumes of fragmented inputs that enter the system without stabilization, forcing rapid interpretation and compressing processing into incomplete pathways. This degrades structure over time. Rebuilding cognition restores control at each stage of transformation so that inputs are processed through a consistent, repeatable framework rather than through reactive approximation.

The process begins with input stabilization. Each incoming signal is decomposed into explicit variables before any reasoning occurs. Terms that carry multiple meanings are separated into distinct components with fixed boundaries. This prevents ambiguity from entering the system and ensures that all subsequent transformations operate on defined elements. Without this step, the system processes shifting representations, producing outputs that vary depending on interpretation rather than structure.

Relationship reconstruction follows. The system re-establishes how variables interact under specific conditions, replacing pattern-based associations with explicit mappings. Each interaction is defined in terms of direction, magnitude, and dependency, allowing the system to execute transformations that can be tested against observed outcomes. This replaces narrative-driven reasoning with controlled state transitions, ensuring that outputs emerge from defined pathways rather than from surface coherence.

Constraint enforcement is reintroduced to limit valid states. Each variable and relationship operates within boundaries that define what configurations are possible. These constraints are applied at every step, preventing the system from generating outputs that rely on invalid intermediate states. Rebuilding cognition requires restoring these boundaries because their absence allows the system to drift into internally consistent but externally invalid conclusions.

Sequencing discipline restores continuity. Transformations are ordered so that each step builds on a correctly defined intermediate state. The system resists compression of sequences, ensuring that no step is skipped or rearranged to accelerate output. This preserves traceability, allowing each conclusion to be linked back through a complete chain of transformations. Without sequencing integrity, the system cannot reliably identify where errors occur or how to correct them.

Feedback integration reconnects the system to reality. Each execution produces a comparison between predicted and observed states, revealing where the model diverges. These deviations are localized and used to refine specific components of the architecture. Over time, this process reduces the gap between internal representation and external conditions, allowing the system to maintain alignment across varying inputs.

Removal of reactive overrides stabilizes processing. Emotional and contextual pressures that previously altered variable weighting or bypassed constraints are isolated and treated as explicit inputs rather than as modifiers of the entire system. This prevents transient states from altering the structure of reasoning, ensuring that outputs remain consistent regardless of internal or external pressure.

Rebuilding cognition therefore transforms the system from a reactive processor into a controlled architecture. Inputs are stabilized, relationships are defined, constraints are enforced, and sequences are preserved. Each execution contributes to refinement through feedback, allowing the system to improve its alignment with the environment over time. The result is a form of thought that operates through structure rather than through approximation, producing outputs that remain consistent, traceable, and adaptable across conditions.

Chapter 27

Final Positioning

Final positioning is the state in which the system operates from a stable, self-reinforcing architecture that consistently produces aligned outputs across conditions. It is not a fixed endpoint or a completed model. It is a configuration where variables remain defined, relationships are applied correctly, constraints are enforced without exception, and sequencing is preserved under pressure. The system no longer relies on intermittent correction or external guidance to maintain alignment. It sustains its own structure through continuous execution and feedback integration.

The positioning begins with structural consolidation. Components that have been refined through repeated cycles are no longer treated as provisional. Variable definitions are fixed within bounded ranges, eliminating ambiguity at the point of entry. Relationships are encoded with explicit conditions, preventing misapplication across different states. Constraints are enforced as non-negotiable boundaries, removing invalid pathways before they can influence output. Sequencing becomes automatic, with transformations applied in the correct order without requiring reconstruction. This consolidation reduces variability and ensures that each execution begins from a consistent baseline.

Operational consistency defines the system's behavior. The same input processed through the same architecture produces the same output, regardless of context or internal state. This repeatability allows the system to scale because outputs can be predicted and extended across larger sets of inputs. Variability is no longer introduced by the system itself. It originates only from changes in input conditions. This separation allows the system to isolate external variation from internal instability, maintaining control over its processing.

Adaptive stability allows the system to evolve without losing coherence. Continuous feedback integration ensures that deviations are detected and corrected at the component level, while constraint enforcement prevents modifications from introducing contradictions. The system changes where necessary but preserves its structural integrity. This balance allows it to remain aligned across new conditions without requiring complete reconstruction of its architecture.

Efficiency is embedded within the structure. Redundant transformations have been removed through iterative refinement, and valid pathways are executed with minimal overhead. The system does not achieve speed by bypassing steps. It achieves speed by organizing its operations so that only necessary transformations are performed. This produces outputs with lower resource cost while maintaining accuracy and reliability.

Transfer capability defines the system's reach. Because variables, relationships, and constraints are encoded at an abstract level, the system can map new inputs onto its existing architecture. This allows it to operate across domains without rebuilding its model. Each new context becomes an extension of the same structure rather than a separate problem space. This reduces adaptation cost and increases the system's ability to maintain alignment in unfamiliar conditions.

Self-monitoring maintains positioning over time. The system continuously checks for consistency across executions, detecting when identical inputs produce divergent outputs or when similar structures yield different results. These signals indicate structural instability, prompting immediate localization and correction. This prevents drift and preserves the integrity of the architecture as it evolves.

Final positioning therefore represents a system that has achieved control over its own operation. It processes inputs through a stable, self-correcting architecture that maintains alignment, consistency, and efficiency across conditions. The system is not static. It continues to evolve through feedback, but it does so within a framework that preserves coherence. This positioning creates a sustained advantage because outputs remain reliable, adaptable, and scalable, reflecting the accumulated refinement of the system's internal structure.

The Future Belongs to Thinkers

Advantage accumulates in systems that control how inputs are transformed rather than in systems that simply receive more inputs. As information volume increases, unstructured processing saturates. Additional data introduces noise, conflicting signals, and inconsistent outputs because the system lacks a stable method for organizing and transforming what it receives. Structured systems operate differently. They convert inputs into defined variables, apply consistent relationships, enforce constraints, and preserve sequencing. This allows them to absorb increasing volumes of information without degradation. Output quality improves with scale because the architecture filters, organizes, and executes transformations in a controlled manner.

Amplification begins with reuse of structure. Once variables, relationships, and constraints are defined and validated, they can be applied across multiple inputs without reconstruction. Each new input passes through the same architecture, producing outputs that are consistent and traceable. This reuse multiplies the effect of each refinement. A single improvement to the structure influences all future processing, increasing overall system performance without requiring additional effort for each instance.

Integration with external systems extends this amplification. When structured reasoning is connected to tools that increase processing speed or expand input access, the architecture determines how effectively those tools are used. A system with weak structure amplifies its errors when given more capacity. A system with strong structure amplifies its accuracy because each additional input is processed through a validated framework. The interaction between structure and capacity defines the rate at which advantage grows.

Feedback-driven refinement accelerates amplification. Each execution generates data that can be used to improve the architecture. As the system processes more inputs, it encounters a wider range of conditions, exposing limitations in its variables, relationships, and constraints. These limitations are corrected and integrated, improving the structure. Because the refined structure is reused across all future processing, each correction produces a multiplied effect. The system improves faster as it processes more data, creating a feedback loop between scale and accuracy.

Constraint enforcement maintains control during amplification. As the system scales, the number of possible pathways increases. Without constraints, this expansion leads to instability and error. Structured systems limit this expansion by restricting transformations to valid states, ensuring that increased processing capacity does not introduce invalid outputs. This containment allows the system to scale without losing alignment.

Sequencing integrity preserves causality under load. Increased throughput creates pressure to compress processing steps. Structured systems resist this by maintaining the order of transformations, ensuring that each output is derived from a complete and valid sequence. This preserves traceability, allowing the system to identify and correct errors even as processing volume increases.

Transferability expands the domain of amplification. Because the architecture operates on abstracted components, it can be applied to new contexts without rebuilding the model. Each additional domain increases the range of inputs that can be processed through the same structure, further multiplying the effect of each refinement. The system's capability grows not only within a domain but across domains, increasing its overall reach.

The boundary between systems becomes more pronounced as amplification progresses. Unstructured systems experience diminishing returns as additional inputs produce inconsistent outputs. Structured systems experience increasing returns because each input contributes to refinement and each refinement improves all subsequent processing. This divergence creates a widening gap in performance that reflects differences in architecture rather than differences in input volume.

The future therefore favors systems that maintain control over their structure. Amplification through structure allows them to convert increasing input and processing capacity into aligned, reliable outputs. Over time, this produces a compounding advantage where each refinement strengthens the system's ability to operate at scale, adapt to new conditions, and maintain consistency across all forms of input.

Thinking as Long-Term Advantage

Long-term advantage emerges when the system's reasoning architecture improves faster than the environment changes. The system does not rely on isolated correct decisions. It relies on a structure that produces aligned decisions consistently, integrates feedback from each execution, and retains those refinements so that future processing begins from an improved state. Positioning is sustained when this cycle operates continuously, allowing the system to adapt without losing coherence and to accumulate improvements that persist across time.

The foundation is structural retention. Each refinement to variables, relationships, constraints, or sequencing is embedded into the model so that it influences all subsequent decisions. This converts short-term accuracy into long-term capability. A system that fails to retain these refinements must solve the same problems repeatedly, preventing accumulation. Sustained positioning depends on converting each resolved deviation into a permanent change in how the system operates.

Consistency across execution stabilizes advantage. The system processes similar inputs through the same pathways, producing predictable outputs that can be evaluated and improved. This repeatability allows feedback to be applied precisely because the relationship between input, transformation, and output remains fixed. Systems that lack consistency cannot accumulate improvement because each execution differs, preventing direct comparison and targeted correction.

Feedback integration drives ongoing alignment. Each decision produces a comparison between predicted and observed states, revealing where the model diverges from reality. These deviations are localized and corrected at the component level. Over time, this reduces error and increases precision. The system does not remain static. It continuously updates its structure to reflect current conditions, maintaining alignment as those conditions change.

Constraint enforcement preserves validity. As the system evolves, it must ensure that new modifications do not introduce states that violate boundaries. Constraints act as a control mechanism, limiting the range of possible transformations and preventing instability. This allows the system to expand its capability without degrading the reliability of its outputs.

Transferability extends advantage across domains. The same architecture can be applied to different contexts by mapping new inputs onto existing variables and relationships. This reduces the cost of adaptation and allows the system to maintain performance as it encounters new conditions. Each domain becomes an additional source of feedback, further refining the model.

Efficiency gains compound over time. As the system refines its structure, it removes redundant transformations and reduces the number of steps required to produce an output. This increases throughput without sacrificing accuracy. The system becomes faster because it is more organized, not because it bypasses necessary processing.

Resilience emerges from continuous correction. When conditions shift, the system detects deviations and adjusts its structure rather than relying on outdated pathways. This prevents large-scale failure by addressing misalignment early. The system maintains function under variation because it is designed to update itself in response to change.

Sustained positioning therefore depends on a system that retains improvements, applies them consistently, integrates feedback continuously, and enforces constraints as it evolves. Thinking becomes an advantage not because of isolated insight, but because the architecture that produces those insights improves with use. Over time, this creates a stable trajectory where each decision contributes to a more accurate, efficient, and adaptable system, maintaining alignment across changing conditions.

Made in the USA
Monee, IL
05 November 2026

67914379R00167